The Simple 0-to-10 GI Diet

The Simple

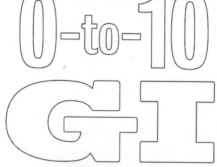

0-to-10

GI

Diet

Lose Weight with the Easy Food-Scoring System Based on the Glycemic Index

AZMINA GOVINDJI BSc RD AND **NINA PUDDEFOOT**

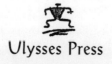

Ulysses Press

Published in the United States by
Ulysses Press
P.O. Box 3440
Berkeley, CA 94703
www.ulyssespress.com

First published as *The GI Plan* in the United Kingdom in 2004 by Vermilion, an imprint of Ebury Press Random House UK Ltd

Printed in Canada by Transcontinental Printing

1 3 5 7 9 10 8 6 4 2

ISBN 1-56975-467-5
Library of Congress Control Number: 2005922423

Cover design: Jake Flaherty

Distributed in the United States by Publishers Group West

This book has been written and published strictly for informational purposes, and in no way should it be used as a substitute for consultation with your medical doctor or health care professional. All facts in this book came from medical files, clinical journals, scientific publications, personal interviews, published trade books, self-published materials by experts, magazine articles, and the personal-practice experiences of the authorities quoted or sources cited. You should not consider educational material herein to be the practice of medicine or to replace consultation with a physician or other medical practitioner. The author and publisher are providing you with information in this work so that you can have the knowledge and can choose, at your own risk, to act on that knowledge. The author and publisher also urge all readers to be aware of their health status and to consult health professionals before beginning any health program, including changes in dietary habits.

The following trademarks are mentioned in *The Simple 0-to-10 GI Diet*, the book is not endorsed by any of the trademark owners: Ryvita is a registered trademark of Associated British Food; Grape-Nuts is a registered trademark of the General Mills Company; Bran Flakes and Raisin Bran are unregistered trademarks of the Kellogg Company; All Bran, Special K, Cornflakes, Rice Krispies and Nutrigrain are registered trademarks of the Kellogg Company; TWIX®, SNICKERS®, MARS® and M&M's® are registered trademarks of Mars UK and are reproduced with kind permission; Splenda is a registered trademark of McNeil Nutritionals, a Division of McNeil-PPC, Inc.; Shredded Wheat is a registered trademark of Nestle U.K. Limited.

The GIS values were adapted with permission from a table of glycemic indices published by the *American Journal of Clinical Nutrition* © Am. J. Clin. Nutr. American Society for Clinical Nutrition.

The authors and publishers have made all reasonable efforts to contact copyright holders for permission, and apologize for any omissions or errors in the form of credit given. Corrections may be made in future printings.

Dedicated to ...

As far as I can remember, this is one of the hardest projects I have ever had to undertake. As I look back on my mother's life, it is she who has inspired me to succeed and to be the very best that I can be. Her foresight and courage have been a living example to me. I would like to dedicate this book to my loving mum, Roshan.

Azmina

My love and thanks go to my dear mum, Joan, and my long-suffering partner, Richard, for their unconditional love and support with my writing and teachings.

Thanks to my close-knit circle of friends, too, for their support and keeping my spirits uplifted.

And, to my co-author, Az, my dear friend and business partner, without whom this book would never have happened.

Nina

Acknowledgements

We'd like to say a huge thank you to our special colleague, Smita Ganatra, whose analytical mind and dietetic expertise have contributed to the meticulous development of the GIS system. Various diet and exercise experts have also been part of the team: Dr. Wynnie Chan, Nigel Denby, Kate Arthur, Sue Baic and Rosita Evans.

The real genius behind such a book is the original researcher. We are indebted to Dr. Jenkins and his team; the authors of the GI international tables: Foster-Powell, Holt and Brand-Miller; McCance and Widdowson's *Composition of Foods*; Jill Davies and John Dickerson's *Nutrient Content of Food Portions*; as well as Dr. Tony Leeds and other authors of *The New Glucose Revolution*, which was great bedtime reading! Thanks also to the host of dietitians who shaped our writing by contributing their personal views on the use of GI — they have been a great encouragement.

To our editor, Amanda Hemmings — thank you for offering us the opportunity to share our concepts and work by being able to express them in this book. A big thank you to Julia Kellaway for her patience and attention to detail. And the most special of all, Azmina's husband Shamil and her young children, Shazia and Bizhan, who often stayed up till the early hours of the morning tirelessly supporting the development of the final manuscript.

To each other — as co-authors and dear chums, we consider ourselves so fortunate to have shared this experience, always being an inspiration to one another, especially when times got tough! This is our special thank you to each other for shared patience and belief—we make a rich team and have a lot of fun along the way.

We would also especially like to thank the following people:

- **Smita Ganatra BSc RD**

  Chief dietitian, Central Middlesex Hospital

  For her professional expertise in assisting in the development of the GIS system.

- **Dr. Wynnie Chan BSc PhD RPHNutr**

  Former Nutrition Scientist for the British Nutrition Foundation

  For providing some of the data analysis.

- **Nigel Denby BSc RD**

  Registered Dietitian, Channel 4's Fit Farm

  For his contribution in helping to make this diet more suitable for men and assisting with the scientific reviews.

- **Kate Arthur BSc RD**

  Registered Dietitian and Sports Accredited Dietitian

  For her contribution to some of the chapters.

- **Sue Baic BSc RD**

  Registered Dietitian and Lecturer in Nutrition at Bristol University

  For providing some of the data analysis.

CONTENTS

TESTIMONIALS FROM DIETERS

The first thing I thought when I browsed through the book was "I can do this. I can do this." The GIS tables covered so many of my usual foods, I could see how easy it was to stick with. I spent the weekend reading through the book more thoroughly, and then I made my shopping list. Having the right foods accessible has been the key.

My best learning so far is the v,v,p,c, which I memorize as "veggie veggie protein carbs." I keep a picture of that plate in my mind when I go to restaurants. I chose a lasagna the other day and the menu said I could have fries or new potatoes, and a vegetable or salad. When I thought about v,v,p,c, I could see that my pasta was the carb, beef was the protein, and I needed to choose the veggie and the salad to get it right. It filled me up, it was delicious and I was keeping to the eat a rainbow guidelines at the same time. When I eat a sandwich, I use the bread as the carb, the filling as the protein, and I make sure I always have a salad (in the sandwich or as extra) as well as a fruit for the veggie portion.

Caroline

I have found it a great help. I have realized that even when I have days when I feel I have slipped a bit, I am making much better food choices without even thinking about it! I am enjoying the snacks and look forward to them without feeling guilty, especially when people at work keep asking "Are you eating again?" I can't thank you enough for bringing me this plan because I don't feel I am going without anything and my meals and my low energy levels are a thing of the past! My skin looks so much better too.

Christine

The best thing about this diet is I don't feel hungry. Normally the minute I start a diet, it feels like I've been on it for a month already. I feel like devouring the most calorific, sugary and fatty cheese cake out there. Now for the first time, I don't feel like I'm on a diet. In fact, *The Simple 0-to-10 GI Diet* forces me to have a snack when I wouldn't normally have one. That's what's helped me to cut down the chips and chocolates on my way home from work. And I'm not known for my self-discipline! I've even replaced late night TV binge-snacking with other tasty and healthier snacks.

Paul

Commitment

Until one is committed there is hesitancy, the chance
    to draw back,
always ineffectiveness.
Concerning all acts of initiative (and creation)
there is one elementary truth,
the ignorance of which kills countless ideas
and splendid plans:
that the moment one definitely commits oneself,
then Providence moves too.
All sorts of things occur to help one
that would otherwise never have occurred.
A whole stream of events issues from the decision,
raising in one's favor all manner
of unforeseen incidents and meetings
and material assistance,
which no man could have dreamt
would have come his way.

Goethe

INTRODUCTION

Congratulations! By picking up this book you've made that all-important first step towards becoming the thinner, healthier, happier "you" that *you* want to be. *Why? Because* the Simple 0-to-10 GI Diet *really works.* (We call it the Simple GI Diet for short.)

What are the three main reasons why dieters give up with other diet plans?

Number 1 — hunger. You just never feel satisfied.
The Simple GI Diet provides **all the food you need** to satisfy your hunger. We even order you to **eat snacks between meals**!

Number 2 — boring foods. You have to eat the very things you don't like.
The Simple GI Diet lets **you eat normal foods**. You choose the foods you like. Just keep to the generous portions and daily allowance and you'll lose weight. And if you go crazy occasionally — hey, that's allowed too!

Number 3 — sticking with it. Who wants to feel they're on a permanent diet?
The Simple GI Diet helps you stay on track with its

tried and tested motivational tools. You're not "on a diet" — you're changing your life, for the better, for good.

So, what's the secret? It includes strategies that *keep you focused* and *keep you full*. If you haven't had much success with other diets, then be prepared to succeed this time, with flying colors. Boost your self-esteem: you can achieve the goals you seek — today, now.

Follow the quick tips and guidelines and see the results for yourself — in your clothes, in your new-found confidence and in the flattering comments of friends, family and partner. Eating the foods you like while watching the pounds slide away and your waist reappear has never been so easy.

And here's a great bonus. You don't have to read the whole book before you get going. Just turn to our Quick Start Guide on page 1 and you can begin the Simple GI Diet today, and take your first step towards becoming the person you want to be. Then, over the next few days, you can take your time to read through this book and discover how and why the Simple GI Diet really works. This is our little gift for you. The Simple GI Diet is your *big gift* to yourself!

This diet is about eating well. Chapter 9 is your comprehensive guide to balanced nutrition. Here are the main benefits in a nutshell. The Simple GI Diet ...

● is simple, practical and flexible. It fits into your

lifestyle—not the other way around.

- uses a blend of the latest scientific knowledge and traditional wisdom to ensure you eat healthily— and still lose weight.
- shows you how to avoid hunger pangs by eating the "right carbs."
- teaches you how to deal with emotional eating and other dieting hurdles—effortlessly!
- helps you become—and stay—motivated, by using insights that tap into the incredible power of your mind.

The result? You reach your target weight and size. And stay there!

NOTE: Glycemic Index is an international ranking of foods, comparing the speed at which a particular food raises blood glucose levels. The Simple GI Diet is designed specifically to take into account the glycemic index and calorie density of foods, and encourages good nutrition.

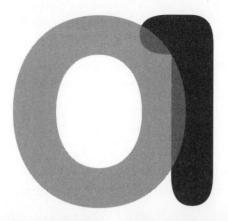

QUICK START GUIDE

So you want to get started right away? Then you've come to the right place since this Quick Start Guide is designed for that purpose. However, it is essential that you read the rest of the book to ensure you are following the plan correctly.

"A good beginning makes a good ending," so the old proverb says. So we believe that a *great* beginning is bound to make a *great* ending. Give this short section your complete attention for the next few minutes—in particular the section entitled "Five crucial minutes towards your goal" (page 4)—even if you're just browsing through this book. Ready?

The low-down on carbs

When you eat "carbs" — or carbohydrate foods (such as bread, potatoes, pasta, cereals and sugary foods), the body digests it and converts it to glucose (a simple sugar). This raises the glucose level in your blood. Different carbs cause the blood glucose level to rise at different rates. Some cause a sharp rise in your blood glucose while others cause a gradual rise.

The Glycemic Index (GI)

The Glycemic Index (GI) is a way of ranking foods based on the rate at which they raise blood glucose levels. Each food is given a number:

- Foods that raise blood glucose quickly have a high glycemic index number. They are best kept to a minimum.
- Foods that raise blood glucose more slowly have a low glycemic index number. These can help you lose weight because they make you feel full for longer.

Keeping your blood glucose levels more stable can improve your sensitivity to an important hormone in the body called insulin. People who are overweight may be less sensitive to insulin, which makes them more prone to diabetes and possibly heart problems.

High-GI foods aren't necessarily bad foods. Neither are low-GI foods necessarily good foods. It is

well recognized that knowing the GI alone is not suffi-
cient for all-around healthy dieting. Hence the Simple
GI Diet.

The Simple GI Diet

The key to successful weight loss is to get the right
mix of foods that ensure stable blood glucose levels
and take into account the calorie value of foods, while
still providing the nutrients needed for optimal
health. This is the unique feature of the Simple GI
Diet. It does all the fancy calculating for you. This
program is an innovative way to choose the right
carbs and stay in shape. It also boasts some of the best-
kept motivational secrets and will-power boosters, as
you'll see throughout the book.

What's the difference between the Simple GI Diet
and a low-carb diet? Lots. But, in a nutshell, the
Simple GI Diet is about choosing the right carbs; those
carbs that are known to be healthy, like wholegrains,
legumes (including peas, beans and lentils), pasta,
fruit and vegetables. In contrast, you get little of these
on a low-carbohydrate diet. The Simple GI Diet
encourages a wide variety of foods so that you are not
missing out on key nutrients. Low-carb diets appear
to restrict certain food groups. The Simple GI Diet
encourages slow, steady and sustainable weight loss
rather than rapid weight loss.

We have given many common food items a certain

number, which we are refer to as the GI Score, or GIS. These are listed in special tables in the book. Each day you have a certain number of GISs that you can use on the foods you want. You choose the foods, so you are in control of what you eat. You just need to follow certain guidelines and keep close to your allocated GISs each day. In no time, you'll learn how to make your GISs go further by choosing wisely, so you lose weight without going hungry. And that's basically it. All you do then is tweak here and there, as you get toward the new slimmer, trimmer and fitter you!

Five crucial minutes toward your goal

Think of a time when you really enjoyed yourself … a vacation perhaps, a party, a sports event or just a good night out. Okay? Now, in your mind, go back in time to that occasion … And as you step into that place, take a moment or so to be there again … Listen to the sounds—what do you hear? What pictures are you seeing? What are you feeling? Enjoy these feelings for a few seconds …

Your mind makes sense of your reality through pictures, sounds and feelings, as we have just seen. Tastes and smells are important too. How does this help you to achieve your goal—for example a slim, trim, new you? Once your goal is clear, your attention automatically focuses on what you need. Your mind selects what it considers to be important in order to achieve the goal. This may include healthier food choices and physical activity as part of your everyday routine. Your energy flows where your attention goes. So what you think about, you bring into your life.

Let's now use this for your specific goal.

What is your goal or outcome?

Take a moment and answer this question as clearly as you can. And here's a big tip—state it in positive words, as something you want rather than something you don't want. Perhaps you really want to get into that bikini, or into your wedding dress. Maybe you want a flatter belly, perhaps a six-pack, or to drop a size, or simply to become trimmer and fitter. Whatever it is, take this time now and answer the question—what is your goal?

Now picture yourself as the person you want to become—the new you. How would you look? Imagine how you would be ... Healthy, fit, energetic, confident? What would you sound like? Be specific. What would you be saying? And how are you saying it? What are others saying about you? Hear their compliments. Connect with your new self now, give yourself a taste of what's to come ... And how are you feeling? Really step inside the new you and experience the feeling. Stay there for a few moments and enjoy it ...

We know from highly successful people that the

A mentor once said:
"I don't start a task until I have decided what the end result is."

goal then becomes just a formality. Now you too have decided what your end result is.

You are a human being, but it's easy to become influenced by others and get busy with too much stuff, which turns you into a human doing! Before you know it, you can lose the plot and fit into somebody else's lifestyle. Now's the time to make different, inspiring choices, to live the life **you** really want, which is lurking within.

How are you feeling now? With your new, inspiring goal fresh in your mind? Please write your goal down as recommended in Step 1 below.

Congratulations, you are now formally in the program.

The Simple GI Diet in 15 steps

Follow these steps and check them off as you get them done.

Step 1: *Write down your goal and the date for reaching that goal.* The best way to keep to a healthy happy weight in the long term is to lose around two pounds each week, so be realistic and your target weight is yours forever.

Also decide how you will know when you've achieved your goal. It may be something you see, something you say or something you hear from others. Or it could be how you feel. Put your goal up somewhere prominent so you can look at it often.

Step 2: *Weigh yourself either now or in the next couple of days.* Check out the BMI chart (page 45) to find a healthy weight for you. There are a couple of other vital measurements that would help you, such as waist measurements. If you want to know about this, turn to page 46. But now let's start to shed some pounds!

Step 3: *Enter the Start-it Phase* (first two weeks). The Simple GI Diet is split into three phases. Each has been carefully designed to guide you to your desired goal in an optimum way. It is important that you follow the instructions to reach your target weight and stay there. You are now starting the first phase of the Simple GI Diet—the Start-it Phase. This is designed to kick-start your weight loss, and is only suitable for the first two weeks. You are likely to lose weight reasonably quickly in this phase, but this initial weight loss is mostly water.

Step 4: *What's my daily allowance?* Use the table below and find the number of GISs you can have per day in the Start-it Phase. You are allowed to have food worth this many GISs each day (for more information on the point system, see page 32).

GISs per day

	Start-it Phase (initial 2 weeks)	Lose-it Phase (until target)	Keep-it Phase (staying on target)
Women	17	20	23 or more
Men	22	25	28 or more

Plus, in addition to your daily GISs, you can have seven ounces of 2% milk each day. What's more, if you want a cocktail, a glass of wine or a beer, that's fine within limits. On the Simple GI Diet, women can include seven alcoholic drinks each week, and men 10 drinks per week (for more on alcohol, see page 119).

Step 5: *Follow the guidelines.* The Simple GI Diet includes some basic guidelines. They are designed to help you lose weight, keep feeling full and get a wide variety of nutrients needed for overall good health. Some are non-dietary—this isn't just a diet, it's a healthy way to be. The complete Simple GI Diet rules are listed at the end of this chapter. Copy and display them in a prominent place. Put them on, say, the fridge door or on your desk at work, so you can look at them often until they become second nature.

Step 6: *Eat three meals and three snacks every day* (**Simple GI Diet Rule 1**). Try to have your main meal at lunchtime and a lighter meal in the evening. Here are a couple of examples of an ideal day during the Lose-it Phase:

<u>Women</u>		<u>Men</u>	
(20-GISs-a-day plan)		(25-GISs-a-day plan)	
Breakfast	4 GISs	Breakfast	5 GISs
Mid-morning	1 1/2 GISs	Mid-morning	2 GISs
Lunch	6 GISs	Lunch	8 GISs
Mid-afternoon	1 1/2 GISs	Mid-afternoon	2 GISs
Dinner	5 GISs	Dinner	6 GISs
Evening snack	2 GISs	Evening snack	2 GISs

Step 7: *Stock up on basic low-GIS foods.* Use our Smart Shopping lists (see pages 55-60) to help you choose. Having these foods handy will make it much easier to enjoy the diet early on. So just photocopy some of the shopping pages and stop at the supermarket on your way home.

Step 8: *Start simple — use the ready-made meal/menu plans provided* (pages 83-96). You might also like to sample the recipes (see pages 126-145). Their GISs are given alongside so you don't have to figure them out. There are meal plans for:

● Breakfasts
● Light and main meals
● Snacks

Or make up your own meals from the GIS Table (see pages 190-227). Or mix and match between the menu plans and the table. It's all about flexibility.

Step 9: *Stay as close as you can to your daily GISs* (**Simple GI Diet Rule 2**). Don't use up all your GISs by lunchtime! Balance your GISs—you'll soon be an expert at budgeting your daily allowance so you're not in the red before sunset. If at times you think you may have a high-GIS meal, then mix a low-GIS carb with it, such as salad, to bring down the overall Glycemic Index of your meal (see page 24). GI research doesn't include all foods so sometimes there is no GIS value. Keep such choices to a minimum.

Step 10: *Have one "meal carb" at each meal, and 2–3 servings of protein each day* (**Simple GI Diet Rule 3**). Meal carbs are carbohydrate foods that have some starch. They are clearly marked in the GIS Table. You need them because this diet is not a "low-carb" diet, it's a "right-carb" diet. Choose 2–3 servings of protein foods (such as lean meat, fish, eggs, beans), keeping to the amounts suggested in the GIS Table. This will help you to balance your meals and maintain Simple GI Diet Rule 5 (see Step 12) at the same time.

Step 11: *Picture your plate in quarters and fill two quarters with vegetables (v, v), one quarter with protein (p) and one quarter with carbs (c).* Here's how you'll remember this: veggie, veggie, protein, carbs (**Simple GI Diet Rule 4**).

Step 12: *Have at least one low-GIS food at each meal and*

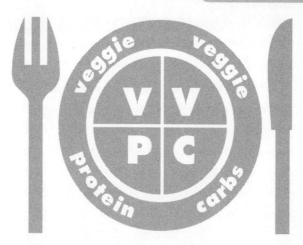

always have a snack (**Simple GI Diet Rule 5**). Making sure you have a snack helps to make the Simple GI Diet work. It keeps that blood glucose level steady and curbs hunger pangs.

Step 13: *Imagine the new you every day — a photograph will help* (**Simple GI Diet Rule 6**). It's not all about what's on your plate. The key is to examine what's going on in your mind.

- *Picture* yourself as the person that you most want to be — the "new" you. See the picture in as much detail as you can, as if it has already happened. See yourself with people who are supportive and fun. See yourself being able to fit into your favorite jeans.
- *Hear* the comments others are making to you, now that you've achieved your goal. Hear their congrat-ulations.

If you are not used to exercise, check with your doctor before you start.

- *Feel* the triumph of your success and how these feelings and emotions make you feel great about yourself. Feel that enhanced sense of energy and inner confidence growing. Put up a photograph of how you want to look—the new you—somewhere you'll see often. That will spur you on even more.

Step 14: *Have at least two 10-minute bursts of moderate-intensity physical activity every day* (**Simple GI Diet Rule 7**). Being GIS-fit means doing only two daily 10-minute bursts of exercise. For example, walk more and walk briskly, use the stairs, get off the bus or subway one stop early and walk, or exercise at home. The possibilities are endless. You could, of course, go swimming, go to the gym, do aerobics, or take up a sport like tennis. Aim at feeling slightly breathless and warm during your 10 minutes of exercise. (But you should not be so breathless that you cannot hold a conversation.)

So decide now what you will do and when. Better to start something small today than wait for something bigger tomorrow. You can always change later. Get someone else to join you if you can.

Step 15: *Choose a balanced diet by having a variety of foods from the different food groups* (**Simple GI Diet Rule 8**).

You can find out more about the food groups in Chapter 9, Eating for Complete Health.

Simple GI Diet Rules

Rule 1: Eat three meals and three snacks every day (page 33).

Rule 2: Stay as close as you can to your daily GISs (page 35).

Rule 3: Have one "meal carb" at each meal, and 2–3 servings of protein each day (pages 38-39).

Rule 4: Picture your plate in quarters and fill two quarters with vegetables (v, v), one quarter with protein (p) and one quarter with carbs (c). Here's how you'll remember this: veggie, veggie, protein, carbs (page 37).

Rule 5: Have at least one low-GIS food at each meal and always have a snack (page 24).

Rule 6: Imagine the new you every day—a photograph will help (page 184).

Rule 7: Have at least two 10-minute bursts of moderate-intensity physical activity every day (page 176).

Rule 8: Choose a balanced diet by having a variety of foods from the different food groups (page 147).

NOTE: These are the basic 15 steps. What next? There are two more things you need to know.

Enter the Lose-it Phase (from week three)

You move on to this phase after the first two weeks. Here you can eat more. Check out the "GISs per day" table on page 8 and read the number of GISs you have per day in the Lose-it column for your gender. You should now have more GISs in a day than before and therefore be able to eat more.

Remind yourself of the 15 steps. Start with the suggested number of GISs, and check your progress at the end of week three. You should be losing one to two pounds per week. Don't be tempted to lose more—research shows that if you try to lose weight too quickly, you are more likely to put the weight back on, as with so many other diets. So keep it slow and steady. Also losing weight too quickly can be harmful to your health in the long term.

Check and correct your daily GISs if appropriate

If you lose more than two pounds per week, increase your daily GISs by 3 or so (you will then eat more and slow down your weight loss).

If you don't lose one to two pounds per week, decrease your daily GISs by 3 or so (you will then eat less and lose more weight).

Having more GISs during the Lose-it Phase simply means you can eat more. Not only does this feel fab, it helps you avoid hunger too. Feeling full and including more daily GISs means that this phase fits more easily into your lifestyle.

Enter the Keep-it Phase

You have reached your target weight. Good job! Reward yourself and enjoy the new you. At this point you enter the Keep-it Phase. Once you've reached a more desirable weight, the GIS system helps you hold on to your new lifestyle. You are in charge of how many GISs you need to keep you thin and fit.

Look at the "GISs per day" table on page 8 and find out the number of GISs you have per day in the Keep-it column for your gender. And use that as your new daily total. Again, check your weight regularly to make sure it's stable. If it's not, adjust your daily GISs a little, as described in the Lose-it Phase. Enjoy!

The key to long-term weight loss: lose 1–2 pounds per week and no more!

Caution

- This chapter gives you just enough information to get you started. It is not designed to give you everything you need. We strongly advise you to read and understand the entire book.

- Be sure to check with your doctor before you start this or any other diet or exercise program.

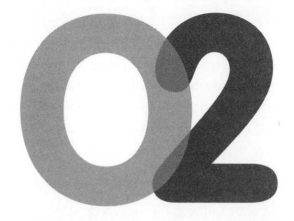

WHAT IS GI?

The carbohydrate controversy

Thumb through any newspaper to see all the conflicting info on carbohydrate foods: "avoid wheat," "starchy foods are fattening," or "pasta is the best food ever invented." How do you know what's best? Well, let's review some of the issues here.

When you eat a carbohydrate food (such as bread, potatoes, pasta, cereals and sugary foods), the body digests it and converts it into glucose (a simple sugar); this can then be used for energy. As the carbohydrate gets converted into glucose, the glucose level in your blood rises.

We know different foods cause the blood glucose to rise at different rates. Some foods cause a sharp rise in your blood glucose levels, and these are best kept to a minimum. Other foods cause a gradual rise in blood glucose levels, and these can help you lose weight. So the speed at which carbohydrate foods are digested plays an important part in losing weight and in over-all health, as we will now see.

The Glycemic Index

The Glycemic Index (GI) ranks foods according to the speed at which they raise blood glucose levels. Each food is given a number:

- Foods that raise blood glucose quickly are said to have a high Glycemic Index.
- Foods that raise blood glucose more slowly have a low Glycemic Index.

Here's a simplified way of looking at this:

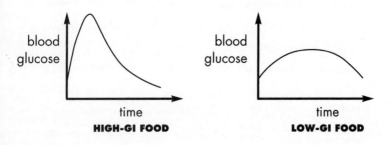

The Glycemic Index has been studied around the world for years and the findings have been published extensively in medical journals (for Research, References and Further Reading see page 228).

Filling not fattening

So how does GI help us? Well, there are two huge benefits. The first good news is for dieters because the more stable your blood glucose levels, the less hungry you will feel.

Foods that cause sharp rises in blood glucose are best kept to a minimum, because they don't fill you up as much, making you more likely to reach for the cookie jar. Foods that cause a rapid rise in blood glucose have a high GI, so the key is to regularly choose more foods with low GIs (we'll see how later).

The main thing to remember is that low-GI foods are digested slowly and cause a slow and steady rise in blood glucose, followed by a steady fall. Slower digestion helps to make you feel full for longer, and so delays hunger pangs. In this book we call these foods the "right carbs."

And here's a bonus—the effect of a low-GI meal can extend to the following meal, which helps keep blood glucose more even throughout the day. This, in turn, helps you control hunger pangs.

This principle, though complex, is based on how you digest food and how a particular food acts within your body to help you feel full for longer.

In 2000, D. S. Ludwig conducted a review of the effects of GI on obesity and concluded that "To date at least 16 studies have examined the effects of GI on appetite and all but one have demonstrated an increase in satiety, delayed hunger return and reduced food intake following low GI foods than following high GI foods" (see Research, References and Further Reading, page 230).

The second benefit of choosing low-GI foods is that foods that raise your blood glucose slowly help to prevent or minimize diabetes and obesity. Research has also shown that people who have an overall low GI diet have a lower incidence of heart disease, and lower GI diets have been associated with improved levels of "good" cholesterol, too.

A lot of this is common sense: "whole" foods, such as wholegrains, and foods high in a particular type of fiber called "soluble fiber," such as kidney beans, take longer to be broken down by the body compared to, say, a soft drink. Therefore grains and beans cause a slower rise in blood glucose. These foods have a relatively low GI. Filling up on low-GI carbohydrate foods during meals and snacks means there's less room for fat, so when you're watching your weight, you're also helping to keep your calorie intake down. The trick is to choose the right carbs rather than avoiding carbs altogether.

It is cumbersome, impractical and not sensible to use the GI in isolation. The Simple GI Diet does all the fancy calculating for you, taking note of the calories and GI, giving you a simple method that you can use with confidence.

So, is it simply a matter of knowing your GIs?

The GI only tells you how quickly or slowly a food raises blood glucose. But foods with a high GI are not bad foods. Compare potato chips, which have a medium GI, to a baked potato, which has a high GI. Interestingly, white pita bread has a lower GI than whole wheat bread—could you ever have guessed that? And some cookies, crackers and cakes have a lower GI than bread—does this mean we should fill up on these?

The key to using GI successfully in weight loss is to get the right mix of foods. This will not only ensure more stable blood glucose levels, it will also take into account the calorie value of the foods and help you obtain the wide variety of nutrients needed for overall good health. This is the unique feature of the GIS system. It is a revolutionary way to choose the right carbs and stay in shape forever. This diet program has another plus—it is supported by some of the best-kept motivational secrets and will-power boosters.

Let's take another example. Chocolate has a medium GI—so does this mean you can have your cake and eat it too? As always, there is a place for

Tip: Keep starchy foods as whole as possible; avoid mashing or processing them since this can raise the GI.

chocolate, though it's advisable to limit it to small amounts at the end of a high-fiber meal. The fiber helps to slow down digestion. Chocolate may have a low GI, but since it's also a high-fat, high-calorie food, this isn't the way the Glycemic Index was intended to be used. Choosing foods with a low GI—as well as those that are low in saturated fat—makes good sense. And since we eat meals, not single foods, eating mainly low-GI foods along with a few high-GI foods will ensure you're being practical and realistic and yet keeping to an overall medium GI in your diet.

Are carbs cool—or not?

It was once believed that all starchy carbohydrate foods, such as bread, rice and potatoes, were digested slowly, causing a gradual increase in blood glucose levels. However, it is now known that many starchy foods, such as certain types of rice and bread, are digested very rapidly and absorbed quickly. They are high-GI carbs.

There are some foods, such as beans and lentils, that would seem to have an obviously lower GI. But the way that they are cooked or processed can also affect

In short, some carbs are great and others should probably be substituted with alternatives, even if it's the same basic food, just cooked or prepared differently.

the GI. So, for example, dried kidney beans boiled have a very low GI, but scoop them out of a can and you'll find that the GI reaches a medium classification. An orange has a low GI, but squeezing it into orange juice raises the GI. In contrast, the acids in lime or lemon juice can help to lower the overall GI of a meal. A serving of peeled boiled potato has a medium GI, but make this into mashed potatoes and the GI reaches the "high" category (even higher for instant mashed potatoes). So, the more mashed up or processed a food is, the higher its GI is likely to be. Use the GIS Tables (pages 190-227) to give you a more accurate assessment of how a food will affect your blood glucose levels—and your weight—rather than just guessing.

What, no more high GIs? Ever?

If you only ate low-GI foods, you might lose weight, but you wouldn't stick to it for long. And, as with many other diets, the weight would creep back on again. The key is to enjoy what you eat, choosing foods that fit in with who you are, your lifestyle, your likes and dislikes, and so on. Although foods with a high GI do not offer favorable effects on blood glucose, we're only human. So why deny yourself the occasional high-GI food? Indeed these foods may be good for you in other ways. Take bread, for example: multigrain bread has a lower GI than other breads, but what if you detest the stuff? Do you go without bread and crave it every time you pass the bakery? Not on the Simple GI Diet, you don't. You make choices based on what else you're eating. You might opt for white bread, a higher-GI food, but then add some baked beans (a medium-GI food) on top to lower the overall blood glucose response.

Meal combos

When you mix foods together in a meal, this affects the GI — and it isn't simply a case of taking the average GI of the individual foods to find out the overall GI of the meal. However, you can predict the GI of a meal using a special formula. The GIS Table has already used this formula to calculate a selection of breakfasts, light meals and recipes for main meals, so you can have a more accurate value for these mixed meals. It would be impossible to calculate all possible meal and food combinations, so use the sample mixed meals as often as you like and mix and match your other food choices with this. The key to remember is to choose low-GIS carbs at each meal or snack. Then you know you're doing the best you can while enjoying variety and freedom of choice.

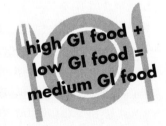

high GI food + low GI food = medium GI food

Can we play the guessing game?

Popcorn has a much higher GI than regular corn. Popcorn is high in fiber and protein and is a great snack food, but because the GI is considered to be high, you'll notice that it's been given more GISs than some other snack foods (see page 205). However, if you do opt for crunching the corn, you could try making your own so that it's not cooked in a lot of oil and smothered in salt. Eating popcorn with a low-GI food, such as nuts, also helps, so long as you're not downing it by the bowlful! (See the recipe for Chili Peanut Popcorn, page 131).

Do all foods have a GI?

No. And since low-GI foods are good choices, you might assume that those with no GI would be better for you—not true. Many non-carbohydrate foods won't raise blood glucose, so they won't have a GI figure. But they might not be good for weight loss. Take fried steak or lard, for example. The Simple GI Diet takes weight loss and good nutrition into account so that you are generally choosing GI-free foods that are lower in fat, especially saturated fat. In this way, you are more likely to choose low GI foods in the right context.

And the calculation of GI requires careful laboratory analysis—not all foods have been analyzed, even if they do contain carbs. Some branded foods, such as Kellogg's All Bran, have been analyzed, but to avoid promoting specific brands, generic names are used in some cases.

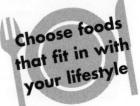

Choose foods that fit in with your lifestyle

Other benefits of the GI way of eating

- Foods that have a low GI are often high in fiber. Choosing those that are low in fat, too, such as pasta, will fill you up and cut down on calories, helping you to maintain a healthy weight.

- People who are overweight and/or have diabetes are more prone to coronary heart disease. A diet based on low- or medium-GI foods, as part of a healthy lifestyle, can be particularly useful in helping to reduce the risk of heart disease for these people. Some low-GI foods, such as those high in soluble fiber (beans, peas and lentils) can also help reduce blood cholesterol.

- People who have a condition called reactive hypoglycemia can incorporate a range of low-GI foods to help stabilize their blood glucose levels.

- The right combination of low- and high-GI foods can help sports performance. Low-GI foods, such as pasta, are great for "carbo-loading" (energy storage) before a sports event, and high-GI foods, such as a glucose drink, provide fast-release carbohydrate, quickly replacing glucose in the bloodstream after an event.

Ten Simple GI Diet tips

1 Have one low-GI food at each meal or snack.

2 Choose breakfast cereals based on wholegrains, such as oats (oatmeal for example).

3 Opt for grainy breads made with whole seeds, barley and oats, instead of white or brown bread.

4 Wheat-based pasta, sweet potatoes and basmati rice are cool—enjoy them regularly and check portion sizes in the GIS Tables (pages 190-227).

5 Dairy foods are low GI and high in calcium—so have reduced-fat milk and low-fat yogurt two or three times a day.

6 Eat more beans, lentils and peas. Toss them into stews and casseroles, or simply spice them up with lemon juice and chili for a snack.

7 Go for whole fruits rather than fruit juices. The lower-GI ones include apples, dried apricots, cherries, grapefruit, grapes, oranges, peaches, pears, plums and firm bananas.

Low-GI foods help you control your appetite by making you feel fuller longer, so you eat less.

A rough guideline: foods high in soluble fiber will have a lower GI; keeping starchy foods whole can reduce their GI; eating veggies keeps the GI low.

8 Under is better than over: choose foods that are under-processed — whole or just cooked — rather than overcooked (such as limp vegetables and mashed potatoes).

9 Go for the fiber fill-up (see page 150). It helps slow the digestion and absorption of starchy foods.

10 Most fruit and vegetables have a low-GI rating, and are low in calories and fat — they are your best friends.

The most important product of your life is you

Learn to nurture and nourish yourself by making healthy choices in the foods you eat and the amount of regular physical activity you do. This is vital in building a caring relationship with yourself. If you don't like yourself, you're less likely to care for yourself, let alone others. Caring for your body will encourage you to put the right foods into it.

The GIS IQ Test

Question:

How do you choose your foods?

Choice 1: I seek out and choose foods with low GISs as often as I can.

Consequently, you are making excellent choices for more steady blood glucose, one of your most important goals.

Choice 2: I make food choices irrespective of whether they're high or low GISs.

Consequently, you are less aware of the effects that different foods have on your blood glucose, making it more difficult to keep within your daily allowance.

Choice 3: I choose more foods that are high in GISs because I like them more.

Consequently, your blood glucose levels are more likely to be unstable, so hunger pangs are more likely to occur.

Results:

Choice 1: Congratulations! Making these kinds of conscious choices will enrich your life by giving you a sense of achievement. This, in turn, is likely to keep you motivated and up-beat in your mental approach and attitude.

Choice 2: Ignorance is mental poverty! This could have direct consequences, preventing you from achieving your goal. Enjoy finding out about the choices that exist and take responsibility for your life and its results. After all, you're in control.

Choice 3: You can start by making different choices today, knowing that this will get you nearer to your ultimate "new you" goal. Short term, many will opt for instant gratification, but this can be at the risk of creating long-term success for themselves. Make up your mind to make the change here and now—and then stick with it.

Summary

- Fill up on low-GI carbs at meals, thereby making less room for fat and helping to keep the calories down.
- Choose "whole foods" that take longer to be broken down by the body.
- The GIS diet facilitates more stable glucose levels, and a calorie-controlled eating plan, integrated into a healthy eating and activity program.

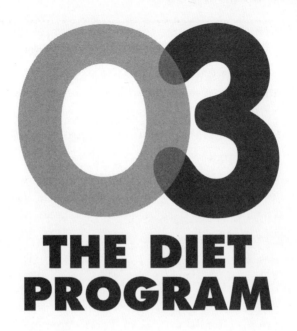

THE DIET PROGRAM

What's so great about GIS?

Dieting using the Glycemic Index alone doesn't necessarily mean you'll lose weight, because you could be filling up on low-GI but high-calorie foods. The Simple GI Diet importantly takes calories into account so that achieving your target weight is all part of the plan.

The beauty of the GIS system is that the experts have done the calculating for you, so all you have to do is add up the GISs you're eating for the day. The system automatically takes into account:

- the Glycemic Index value of the listed foods
- calories

- portion sizes that will fill you up as well as help you lose weight steadily
- healthy eating strategies

This makes the diet healthy, slimming and practical. How easy is that?

GISs uniquely incorporate the Glycemic Index, calories and good nutritional guidelines, which you cannot achieve using the GI alone.

The GIS system

The system is really very easy. Food items have been given a certain number of GISs. Now, imagine that you're given an allowance of GISs each day, which you can spend on the foods you want to eat. Just as you would spend money to buy food from a store, here you choose which foods you spend your GISs on that day. So you are in control of what you eat.

Stay as close as you can to your daily allowance of GISs, and each new day you get another set of GISs to spend. It's just like going to the cash machine.

You'll learn how to make your GISs go further by choosing wisely, so you lose weight without going hungry. What's more, you even get a bonus—you follow some basic tips and you'll even end up having a nutritious and balanced diet without thinking too much about it. So you'll not only lose weight, but you'll also be taking care of that all-important tool in your life—your body.

All this will help you learn new skills and behaviors. They will soon become automatic—actions that you do almost without thinking, like driving a car or swimming. This soon becomes a lifestyle change that lasts forever!

So, are you ready for the new slimmer, trimmer and fitter you? Then let's get started.

GI is based on how foods affect your blood glucose levels so one of the keys to GIS eating is to eat regular meals and snacks. In fact, you're eating six times a day! Simply spread out your GISs to suit your lifestyle and tastes, making sure you distribute them evenly throughout the day. Try to have your main meal at lunchtime and a lighter meal in the evening.

For example, if you are on the 20-GISs-a-day plan (for women), your ideal day might look like this:

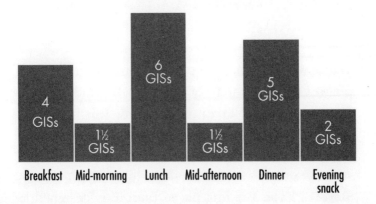

Breakfast	Mid-morning	Lunch	Mid-afternoon	Dinner	Evening snack
4 GISs	1½ GISs	6 GISs	1½ GISs	5 GISs	2 GISs

And a 25-GISs-a-day plan (for men) might look like this.

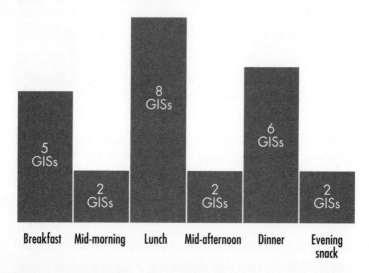

5 GISs	2 GISs	8 GISs	2 GISs	6 GISs	2 GISs
Breakfast	Mid-morning	Lunch	Mid-afternoon	Dinner	Evening snack

Simple GI Diet Rule 1:
Eat three meals and three snacks every day.

The Simple GI Diet phases

Start-it ⇨ Lose-it ⇨ Keep-it

The Simple GI Diet is split into three phases. Each phase has been carefully designed to guide you to your desired goal in an optimal way. It is important that you follow the instructions below to reach your target weight and stay there.

Start-it Phase: The first phase, Start-it, is designed to kick-start your weight loss, but is only appropriate for the first two weeks. During this phase you are likely to lose weight reasonably quickly. As with any weight-loss plan, most of the initial weight loss is just water.

Lose-it Phase: The second phase, Lose-it, allows you more daily GISs. This is designed to help you eat more and lose weight more steadily and sensibly. The ideal rate of weight loss is around one to two pounds per week.

If you opt for fewer GISs, you'll probably lose weight more quickly. But research shows that trying to lose weight too quickly is not effective in keeping the weight off permanently. You are more likely to put the weight back on, as happens with many other diets. So keep it slow and steady, especially since losing weight too quickly can be harmful in the long term.

Keep-it Phase: Once you've reached a more desirable weight, the GIS system helps you hold onto of your new lifestyle. You are in charge of how many GISs you need to keep you slim and fit.

How many GISs for me?

In general, women are likely to lose an appropriate and steady amount of weight on 20 GISs per day, and 25 GISs a day is likely to suit men best. Use the table below to figure out your daily GISs. The calories you need to stick to in order to lose weight slowly and successfully depend on your age, weight and activity levels. However, this is a useful starting point for new dieters:

	Start-it Phase (initial 2 weeks) GISs per day	Lose-it Phase (until target) GISs per day	Keep-it Phase (staying on target) GISs per day
Women	17	20	23 or more
Men	22	25	28 or more

Be wise with your GISs

If you gobble a couple of croissants for breakfast (12 GISs), a slice of cake mid-morning (6 GISs), and a hot dog with mustard at lunch (around 9 GISs), then you know you have already blown it—with nothing left for dinner! The key is to get smart by balancing your GISs. You'll soon be an expert at budgeting your daily GISs so that you're not maxed out before dinner. Get into the habit of checking that you have enough GISs left for dinner and the rest of the day.

Many meals and snacks (for example, those eaten at breakfast, mid-morning and lunch) become habitual. Our choice of foods for these three eating sessions are often very similar. So it's likely that you will soon get to know how many GISs you have left for the

Simple GI Diet Rule 2:
Stay as close as you can to your daily GISs.

evening. You might choose to have a different distribution of GISs on the weekend, which is okay.

Since the goal is to keep your blood glucose levels more or less steady throughout the day, having a rough guide to the number of GISs per meal or snack can be very helpful.

There will be times when only a high-GIS meal will do — and that's fine. Simply mix in a low-GIS carb (see page 24). This helps you to lower the overall glycemic effect of the meal (for more on this, see Chapter 2). And if on occasion you don't know the GIS value of a meal, watch your portion size and add a low-GIS carb to it, just as a safeguard.

Picture your plate

Remember Simple GI Diet Rule 4: *Picture your plate in quarters.* Two parts are to be filled with veggies and/or salad, one with meat, fish, legumes, etc., and the last quarter with starchy food like potatoes, pasta or rice.

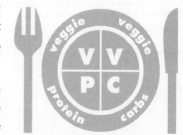

In this way, you will instinctively be keeping to healthier proportions. Try thinking of meals as two veggies plus meat, rather than meat and two veggies. The vegetables are best treated as an integral part of the meal. Having your plate piled up with veggies and salad is a great way to make sure you get a range of vitamins and minerals. You'll also find that most of these foods are either GIS-free or very low in GISs, so they'll fill you up and keep you trim. When it comes to carbohydrates, base meals and snacks on low-GIS carbs. Pasta and grainy breads fill you up and have a lower GI, so choose them often.

Choose a balanced diet

Remember Simple GI Diet Rule 8: *Choose a balanced diet by having a variety of foods from the different food groups.*

Any dieting plan must encourage an overall balance of healthy foods. Details of the different food groups and nutrients are dealt with in Chapter 9—Eating for Complete Health. For now, use the following guidelines as a checklist to make sure you get the balance right. Each day:

● Eat three meals and three snacks; keep fatty and sugary choices to a minimum.

GIS Rule 5:
Have at least one low-GIS carb at each meal and always have a snack.

- Have a "meal carb" at each meal.
- Choose two to three portions of protein foods each day (such as lean meat, fish, eggs, cheese and beans), keeping to the amounts suggested in the GIS Table.
- Eat at least five portions of fruit and vegetables.
- Remember to picture your plate in quarters and to fill two quarters with vegetables (v, v), one quarter with protein (p) and one quarter with carbs (c) (veggie, veggie, protein, carbs).
- Drink six to eight glasses of fluid (such as water, low-calorie drinks, herbal teas, milk, tea, coffee).
- Have a free daily allowance of seven ounces of 2% milk (an extra ½ GIS) in addition to milk with your breakfast cereal.
- Alcohol—no more than seven drinks for women and 10 drinks for men per week; this is in addition to your daily allowance (an optional bonus!). It's better to drink less, though, and make sure you distribute your alcohol intake throughout the week.

Forcing yourself to have a snack may seem a bit pointless, but it is one of the foundations of the GIS system. Having a snack between meals helps to keep your blood glucose level steady.

The foods and their GISs

GI only applies to carbohydrate foods. Not all foods have been analyzed by researchers, even if they do contain carbs. So it is not possible to know the GISs of every food. However, the GIS Tables (pages 190-227) include a wide range of everyday foods so you can enjoy variety and flavor at home, at work and when eating out.

Non-carbohydrate foods (such as meat and cheese) have been given a GIS value based on a Glycemic Index of zero, as defined by international research (page 235). You'll note that fatty meats and some other high-saturated-fat foods have not been listed — it's best to keep these to a minimum.

GIS-free foods

There are certain foods that are so low in GISs that you can enjoy them freely. Yes ... they don't count towards your daily allowance — you can have them for free!

You can eat some of these as much as you like, and others have a specified portion size. Check the GIS Table for a large selection of these delights.

Low-GIS carbs

Use these foods to make up your daily GISs whenever possible. By choosing low-GIS foods, you'll get more food for your GISs! Again, check out the GIS Table for details.

What about prepared foods and eating out?

You'll notice that there are some prepared foods in the GIS Table. As mentioned above, if the Glycemic Index of a meal has not been specified by researchers, then we don't know the GIS value. So try to stick to the foods with a value, but use your common sense when you can't. It's far better to eat fresh foods, but there will be days when only food in a box is available and

Vitamins—Who Needs Them?

It is preferable to get our nutrients from natural foods when possible. However, we do live in the real world, with hectic lifestyles, stress, and the availability of packaged meals and takeout. It's not always easy to eat well. You might therefore want to take an all-around vitamin as a safety net, but make sure it provides no more than 100 percent of the recommended daily amount (RDA) of particular vitamins and minerals. If you are tempted by capsules that offer large doses of vitamins or minerals, proceed with caution. Some of these nutrients are stored by the body and can be harmful if taken in excess.

Certain groups, such as pregnant women, diabetics and the elderly, may require particular vitamins and are advised to speak to their doctor.

you won't know the GIS value—just don't go overboard. Try to keep it to once a week, and be sure to mix in a low-GIS food with it, such as vegetables or a salad, to lower the overall glycemic effect.

As for eating out, turn to Chapter 7 for a bunch of GIS tips.

Tips for healthy eating

Here are some helpful tips that encourage you to make small changes to the way you eat, which in turn can help keep you trim. Try one at a time and slowly build up until you can do them all.

- Treat everything you eat as a meal. Sit down, ideally at the dinner table rather than in front of the TV. Sit upright.
- Take a break from whatever you're doing when you choose to have a snack.
- Avoid eating lunch at your desk. And if you do have a snack at the PC, just relax your hands, move back a little and enjoy every mouthful.
- Have planned meals and snacks. If you simply nibble a bit here and there, note that this may influence your blood glucose, so it's better to keep to your three meals and three snacks a day.

You don't need to avoid any food—simply think about how you can make it better. And if you can't, ask yourself whether there's another choice you can make.

● Put your knife and fork down after you've taken a mouthful. It allows time for chewing your food well, having a drink and engaging in conversation. Chewing slowly and eating at a steady pace can also reduce bloating and improve digestion.

What if the weight just falls off?

That's great! Or is it? Weigh yourself once a week — choose a day that suits you. Mondays may not be the best day if you're indulgent on the weekends! You are likely to lose more than two pounds during Start-it, especially if you follow all the Simple GI Diet rules. However, if at the end of week three you are still losing more than two pounds a week, simply add a few more GISs (say, three) until the weight loss becomes more slow and steady. You are the best judge of how many GISs you need for an ideal rate of weight loss. It's best not to get tempted into staying with a low-GIS diet just so that the weight rolls off quickly — you are then less likely to keep the weight off in the long run.

As always, if you're concerned about your weight loss or anything else in your diet, consult your doctor, who may refer you to a dietitian.

What's my target weight?

So you're committed to sticking with the plan and to enjoying your new easy lifestyle that allows you to eat what you like as long as you keep to some basic guidelines. But how do you know what your ideal weight is? And is it more helpful to think of a "happy weight" for you?

Body mass index

The body mass index (BMI) is one technique used by doctors and dietitians to assess whether you are at a healthy weight. To calculate your BMI, take your weight (in pounds) and divide this by your height (in inches) squared, multiplied by 703.

$$\textbf{BMI} = \frac{\textbf{Weight (lbs)}}{\textbf{Height (in)2}} \times \textbf{703}$$

The most desirable range is a BMI of between 20 and 24. A higher BMI is an indication of being overweight.

The BMI chart (opposite) will help you to figure out just how much weight you need to lose to be within a healthy range. Plot your height (without shoes) on the left-hand axis. Plot your weight (without clothes) on the horizontal axis. Make a straight line from each mark and note where the two lines meet. This will show you what your BMI is—your target weight will be in the 20 to 24 range. Aim for the higher end of this range for now. Once you have maintained your new weight for a few months, you

Body Mass Index Chart

Height	Weight											
4'10"	91	96	100	105	110	115	119	124	129	134	138	143
4'11"	94	99	104	109	114	119	124	128	133	138	143	148
5'0"	97	102	107	112	118	123	128	133	138	143	148	153
5'1"	100	106	111	116	122	127	132	137	143	148	153	158
5'2"	104	109	115	120	126	131	136	142	147	153	158	164
5'3"	107	113	118	124	130	135	141	146	152	158	163	169
5'4"	110	116	122	128	134	140	145	151	157	163	169	174
5'5"	114	120	126	132	138	144	160	156	162	168	174	180
5'6"	118	124	130	136	142	148	155	161	167	173	179	186
5'7"	121	127	134	140	146	153	159	166	172	178	185	191
5'8"	125	131	138	144	151	158	164	171	177	184	190	197
5'9"	128	135	142	149	155	162	169	176	182	189	196	203
5'10"	132	139	146	153	160	167	174	181	188	195	202	207
5'11"	136	143	150	157	165	172	179	186	193	200	208	215
6'0"	140	147	154	162	169	177	184	191	199	206	213	221
6'1"	144	151	159	166	174	182	189	197	204	212	219	227
6'2"	148	155	163	171	179	186	194	202	210	218	225	233
6'3"	152	160	168	176	184	192	200	208	216	224	232	240
6'4"	165	163	172	180	189	197	205	213	221	230	238	246
BMI	19	20	21	22	23	24	25	26	27	28	29	30

Step 1: Find your height on the left side of the chart.
Step 2: Follow along to the right until you find your weight.
Step 3: Go straight down from your weight to find your BMI on the bottom line.

can then aim for a lower weight by reducing your GISs, so long as you keep within the healthy weight range—don't go overboard!

Take the backpack test

As you lose weight, whether it's half a pound or two pounds, put an object of the same weight into a backpack or shopping bag. As you continue to lose weight, add other items (such as a box of sugar for every pound) and just see and feel the weight pile up in the bag while it drops off your body.

The "fruit salad" theory

Are you an "apple-shape" or a "pear-shape"?

This may sound unimportant, but in fact sound scientific theories have been formulated using this information. Putting weight on around the tummy, called "central obesity," is said to be associated with resistance to insulin, which in turn has been shown to make you more prone to certain medical conditions. People with a larger waist measurement have a higher risk of diabetes and heart disease.

Here's the low-down. You're in the "watch-out" category if:

● You're a man whose waist measures more than 37 inches.

- You're a woman whose waist measures more than 32 inches.

- You're a man of South Asian origin (such men have been found to be even more at risk) whose waist measures more than 36 inches.

So, getting closer to a pear-shape may actually offer some protection. This is where GIS can help. Choosing foods that are low in GISs and staying with the right number of daily GISs for you, on average, while taking on board the physical activity guidelines (see Chapter 10) can help to reduce excess abdominal fat, getting you into a better body shape. And when you reach your target, phase three (Keep-it) is just the ticket for staying in shape—forever.

Take the tape test

Find an old belt and use some brightly colored tape to mark the section that fits you today. As your waist/belly gets smaller in the coming weeks and months, add more pieces of tape so you can see how well you're doing. Keep the belt for old time's sake— you might need something to prove to your friends what your waist used to look like!

Keeping the weight off

Get to the stage where you want to keep to your healthier eating habits and activity levels, because the pay-off encourages you to keep going. It's all about motivation. You want to stay there because you recognize that the results are greater than they would be if you went back to your old ways. Think about how you got to your target weight and all the benefits this has given you. Write them down and look at your list often. If you have reached your target weight sensibly you won't just have been eating less, you will have changed your shopping and cooking habits too. So set yourself small targets to keep yourself motivated.

Stay slim tips:

● Your Keep-it GIS diet is your new way of life. You may lapse occasionally, that's fine. Just acknowledge it and start again.

● If you put on a pound or two you can always take it off again, so don't punish yourself. Just get back on track.

● Find ways to make your regular routine and your family support you. You are going to *stay* slim and healthy.

- Before you reach for the cookie jar, ask yourself if it's going to take you nearer to the "new" you. If it isn't, walk to the fruit bowl!

- Stay fit with family and friends. It's much more fun to go cycling or swimming or do other sports with other people.

- Keep a daily food and mood diary (see below) so you can see when you indulge and what your emotions are like at that time, for example, boredom, stress, comfort, security, PMS.

- Now that you have reached your target, what are you going to do next? Why not learn a new sport, or take up a new hobby? Better still, as you start your goal, take up a new interest so that your mind has something to occupy itself.

- Treat yourself to some new clothes. Go through your wardrobe and donate your over-sized clothes to charity. If you make an effort to look good, you'll want to stay thin.

- Be specific about your goal. On such and such a date (specify) I will weigh X.

- Each morning, pour your daily allowance of seven ounces of milk into a bottle or container. It's an easy way to keep track of your milk intake. Cereals in the GIS Table already have milk included in their total.

FOOD AND MOOD DIARY

Food fills a physical, not an emotional, need. When you become more aware of the underlying feeling that is causing you to overeat, you are more able to make some changes. Fill in the daily food journal below to highlight the emotional needs that cause you to have a snack attack. Remind yourself, "What would have to happen, that is within my control, for this need to be met in a healthy and functional way?" Before you seek solace in that "naughty but nice food," ask yourself whether this is taking you

Time	Food & Quantity Eaten	Fruit & Veggies	GISs

TOTAL GISs FOR THE DAY

nearer to the "new" you. If it isn't, choose again! (See page 105 for more advice.) Recording what you eat will also help you to check if you are keeping to the GIS rules and, if not, what you might want to adjust next time.

Week Number . . . .
Day/Date. . . . .
Working/non-working day . . . .

motions, e.g. tired, hungry, feeling low	Comments

Getting started

How do I get started? You can start right here, right now!

1 Weigh yourself. And weigh yourself weekly on the same day, wearing similar clothing.

2 Look at the BMI chart to find your target weight.

3 Measure your waist and figure out if you are an "apple" or "pear" shape so you know where you want to be heading.

4 Get on board with the Start-it Phase using the suggested number of GISs for your gender.

5 Optional (but strongly advised): Do the exercise on imagining the new you (see page 184).

6 Stock up on some low-GIS foods using our Smart Shopping tips (see Chapter 4).

7 Display the Simple GI Diet rules in a prominent place so you can look at them often.

8 Move on to the Lose-it Phase after the first two weeks, starting with the suggested number of GISs. Gauge your progress at the end of week three, and increase your allowance by three GISs or so to slow down your weight loss if it's more than two pounds a week.

9 Keep losing it until you reach your target "happy" weight. Slide into the Keep-it Phase, increasing your GISs without increasing your hips until you are maintaining your new weight.

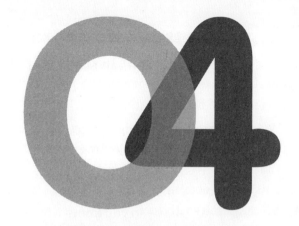

SMART SHOPPING

Walking down the aisle

Whether you're whizzing around the store in 20 minutes, or shopping on the internet, this chapter gives you a speedy low-down on which foods to throw in your shopping cart. And don't worry if you're hooked on supermarket quick fixes, just check out our Food in a Flash section (page 61).

By now you will know that the Simple GI Diet is about eating filling and varied foods—not about specialist health food shopping. There are no aisles in the grocery store to avoid. Here's a trick you can play in order to take home a happy and healthy shopping bag. Imagine your supermarket is divided into five sections representing the main food groups (page 147).

The largest section is at the top and the smallest section is at the bottom:

- Bread, other cereals, such as breakfast cereals, and potatoes.
- Fruit and vegetables.
- Milk and dairy products.
- Meat, fish and alternatives.
- Fatty and sugar-laden foods.

Your cart should contain foods roughly in line with these groups of food. You could even try dividing your time in proportion too. For example, spend more time looking at the variety of fruits and vegetables and high-fiber cereals now available and less time on the smaller sections, like the fatty snack foods. This will help you make healthy choices and will also add variety to your diet. You might find that shopping on the internet saves you money because it stops you from buying foods from less healthy aisles, since you're not tempted by the smells of the bakery or the buy-one-get-one-free offers (probably a food you weren't going to buy anyway!).

Foods that are high in fiber tend to be low in GISs. But that's not always the case, because some high-fiber foods may be loaded with sugar, or they may simply have a higher glycemic value than you'd expect (rice cakes have a high GI for example). So, to keep it simple, just glance at the list below so you know what the usual suspects are going to be. You might like to take a photocopy of these pages with you and highlight what you need that day. You'll soon get to know which foods to grab and which foods to leave on the shelves.

Shopping list of low-GIS foods

Here is a selection of food and drink—choose the ones you like. They are all low in GISs.

Drinks
Coffee, black, no sugar (use milk from your allowance)
Diet soft drinks
Drinkable yogurt
Juice, grapefruit, unsweetened
Juice, orange, unsweetened
Juice, pineapple, unsweetened
Juice, tomato
Milk, reduced-fat
Soy milk, non-dairy alternative to milk, unsweetened
Tea, black, no sugar (use milk from your allowance)
Water, still, sparkling or flavored

Fresh fruit
Apples

Apricots

Melon, cantaloupe

Olives

Bananas
Cherries
Grapefruit
Grapes
Kiwi
Mangoes

Oranges
Peaches
Pears
Pineapple
Plums
Strawberries

Canned fruit

Fruit cocktail, in juice
Peaches, in juice
Pears, in juice

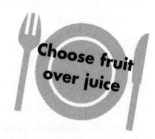

Dried fruit

Apricots
Dates
Figs

Prunes, ready-to-eat
Raisins

Fresh vegetables

Beets
Broccoli
Brussels sprouts
Cabbage
Carrots
Cauliflower
Celery
Celery root
Corn, baby
Corn, on the cob, whole
Cucumber

Fennel
Lettuce
Mushrooms
Plantain
Potatoes
Pumpkin
Rutabaga
Salad vegetables
Sweet potatoes
Yams
Zucchini

Frozen vegetables

Broccoli

Brussels sprouts

Cabbage

Carrots

Cauliflower

Corn, baby or kernels

French beans

Peas

Runner beans

Spinach

Canned vegetables and soups

(Be sure veggies and beans are canned in water; soups should not contain cream.)

Baked beans

Chickpeas

Chili beans

Corn

Kidney beans

Lentil soup

Peas

Instant noodle soup

Minestrone soup

Tomato soup

Cereals

Bran flakes

High-fiber cereals such as All Bran, muesli

Original oatmeal—large-flake variety
Special K

Breads

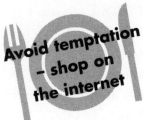

Barley and sunflower bread
Barley bread*
Multigrain bread
Pumpernickel bread
Raisin Bread
Rye bread
Wheat tortillas*
White bread, "with added fiber"

*These have lower GISs compared to the other listed breads.

Dairy
Ice cream, dairy, reduced calorie
Milk, flavored, chocolate, reduced-fat
Milk, 2%
Milk, skim
Soy yogurt, fruit
Yogurt, drinkable
Yogurt, low-fat, plain
Yogurt, virtually fat-free/diet, plain

Pasta
Fettucine, egg
Linguini, thin or thick

Macaroni
Pasta, plain
Spaghetti, white
Spaghetti, whole wheat

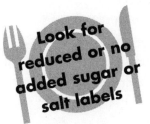
Look for reduced or no added sugar or salt labels

Rice and grains
Barley
Brown rice
Bulgur wheat
Noodles, instant or rice
White rice, Bangladeshi
White rice, basmati

Dried beans and lentils
Black-eyed peas, dried
Chickpeas, split, dried
Chickpeas, whole, dried
Chili beans, dried
Lentils, red, split, dried
Lima beans, dried
Mung beans, whole, dried
Pigeon peas, whole, dried
Pinto beans, dried
Red kidney beans, dried
Soy beans, dried

Miscellaneous
Beets, pickled
Gherkins, pickled

Other regular shopping-basket items
Eggs
Fish
Seasonings (to taste)
Lean meats and poultry
Oil, olive, rapeseed, spray oil (any)

Healthy shopping tips

● Watch out for ever-increasing portion sizes of packaged meals and snacks such as sandwiches, chips and chocolate bars. Just switching from a standard bag of chips to a large bag would lead to a weight gain of over 13 pounds over a year without changing anything else!

● Canned foods such as fruit, vegetables, legumes (beans, peas and lentils) and fish are a useful purchase. Look for those labeled reduced, or no added, sugar or salt.

● Dried and frozen foods are often just as nutritious as fresh, and more convenient if you don't shop often.

● Shop after you've eaten, so it's easier to resist the temptation to buy high-fat, high-sugar foods. Make a shopping list and stick to it.

Many supermarkets provide leaflets on healthy eating and dieting, guiding shoppers to healthy choices. You could also look for a healthy-eating logo, which many major products have. Usually these products will be lower in fat than the standard item and may be lower in calories, sugar and salt, too. But be suspicious of labels boasting "healthy" desserts and cakes—they might be low in fat but high in sugar. This could mean they are not necessarily lower in calories and so are not a great help if you're watching your weight. And remember that a reduced-fat version of a high-fat food isn't a license to grab and go; it could still pile on the fat, so don't go eating twice as much.

Food in a flash

Let's face it, who has the time to cook dinner every night? With today's hectic lifestyles, it's hardly surprising that we get tempted by "microwave in three minutes" or "just stir into cooked pasta" labels. And what's wrong with that? Nothing, if you're a wise Simple GI Dieter. It's all about mix and match. As

Shop wisely!

- Use the shopping list to select those foods that fit in with your Simple GI Diet. Stock up your fridge, freezer and secret snack cupboard with all the goodies that will help you reach your goals.

- See the menu-planning chapter (page 73) for ideas of other foods to buy for the coming week. If, for example, you decide to choose the number 2 meal combo (see page 89), then list the foods that you will need to have at home.

you know, throwing in a low-GIS food will lower the GI of your meal. The good news about the GIS system is that you can still eat convenience foods, so long as you follow some basic guidelines.

If you know the GIS value of the food, you're on your way. Just add it to your daily allowance. If you don't know the GIS value, then:

1 Choose high-fiber versions where possible—many bought foods will be processed, which often makes them lower in fiber than similar products you'd make at home.

2 Choose the right carbs—pita bread instead of French baguette, basmati rice rather than regular white rice, boiled potatoes in their skins instead of instant mashed potatoes.

3 Go for foods that are as close to their "whole state" as you can find, such as chunky tomato pasta sauces. Opt for whole-bean soups, and whole vegetables rather than puréed or creamed versions.

4 Mixing and matching really works—add a low-GIS food, such as salad, your favorite vegetable, grainy bread or a handful of seeds. Or give your meal a low-GI twist by adding a fruity dessert.

5 Check out the fat and calories against your guideline daily amounts (table opposite) and watch out for saturated fats. (See the table on page 68 to get a feel for the numbers for ingredients such as sugar or fat.)

What does the label say?

You just need to scan food labels in your pantry to see that we're bombarded by nutritional information, healthy-eating logos and promotional captions. How on earth do we interpret them, and how do we know which labels to trust? If yogurt has six percent fat, is that a lot, or not? Why is low-fat cheese called that when, in fact, it's a high-fat food? And did you know that some so-called "healthy" granola bars contain as much as 25 percent sugar?

Here's how to tell your "low-fats" from your "fat-frees" and your "no added sugars" from your "sugar-frees."

First, before you interpret the small print, it's helpful to know what you're looking for. Most food labels list Daily Values (DVs). These are guidelines for the average amount of fats, calories and other nutrients recommended in a healthy adult diet. Obviously, they

Daily Values of nutrients for adults*		
Nutrient	**Men**	**Women**
Calories	2500	2000
Total Fat	80 grams	65 grams
Saturated fat	25 grams	20 grams
Cholesterol	300 mg	300 mg
Sodium	2400 mg	2400 mg
Carbohydrate	375 grams	300 grams
Fiber	30 grams	25 grams
*source: www.fda.gov		

are only general guidelines, as your personal needs will vary according to your age, weight, physical activity level, and so on.

Nevertheless, DVs can help you to see whether a particular food might fit into your meals.

Guidelines of common nutrient claims

Nutrition claim	Definition per 100 grams or 100 ml	Example
Low sugar	Contains less than 5 grams of sugar	Low-sugar custard
Low-fat	3 grams of fat	Low-fat rice pudding
Low sodium	40 mg of salt	Low-salt soy sauce
Reduced sugar	Contains 25% less sugar, fat or salt than normal product	Reduced-sugar jams
Reduced-fat		Reduced-fat spreads
Reduced salt		Reduced-salt baked beans
Sugar free	Contains less than 0.2 grams of sugar	Sugar-free jelly Sugar-free soft drinks (may be called "diet")
No added sugar/ unsweetened	No sugars, or foods composed mainly of sugars, have been added to the food	Unsweetened fruit juices

So, looking at the DV guidelines, you know the maximum amounts of fat and so on you need in a day. When you look at the label on a pack of chocolate-chip cookies, you'll notice that you get around 3 grams of fat per cookie. Sounds okay. Add a couple of these to the fat from your cheese and tomato sandwich and bag of chips, and you've scarfed around 30 grams of fat before you've even thought about dinner, or added in what you had for breakfast.

Manufacturers are now starting to use terms on their food labels that have officially recognized meanings. See the chart on the opposite page for an insight.

In the past, manufacturers have sometimes added to the confusion by using "percent fat-free" claims. Think about it—an "85 percent fat-free food" still contains a hefty 15 percent fat! How misleading is that? Nowadays this practice has been more tightly controlled (apart from the quite reasonable "97 percent fat-free" on some products which only contain three percent fat).

You may want to study food labels to help you decide how certain foods fit into your diet, since this helps you to get the most out of the foods you enjoy. This is where reading and understanding the more detailed nutritional information can be a skill worth acquiring. Here's how …

Understanding nutrition information on food labels

The ingredients list will tell you what's in a food but not how much. In this list ingredients appear in descending order of weight, so the first ingredient will be present in the largest quantity and the last ingredient will be the smallest. Before we had nutritional information on labels, this was quite useful. But now the nutritional content is far more relevant. Even if sugar is near the top of the list it doesn't necessarily mean that food is packed with sugar. It all depends on how much of an ingredient is in the package. (Remember, sugar does come in different guises, such as sucrose, dextrose, glucose syrup and maltose.)

To the right is a typical nutrition label.

Let the label be your guide

The Nutrition Facts label on most packaged foods can help you make wise choices. This label for potato chips shows high levels of sodium and fat, low fiber, relatively little carbohydrate and protein, and few vitamins and minerals—except for iron, which you may not want anyway. Probably okay for an occasional treat, but overall not a GIS-friendly food!

Nutrition Facts

Serving Size 1 package
Servings Per Container 1

Amount Per Serving

Calories 230   Calories from Fat 140

	% Daily Value*
Total Fat 15g	**24%**
Saturated Fat 4g	**21%**
Cholesterol 0mg	**0%**
Sodium 270mg	**11%**
Total Carbohydrate 22g	**7%**
Dietary Fiber 1g	**6%**
Sugars 0g	
Protein 3g	

Vitamin A 0%	●	Vitamin C 15%
Calcium 0%	●	Iron 2%

* Percent Daily Values are based on a 2,000 calorie diet. Your daily values may be higher or lower depending on your calorie needs:

	Calories:	2,000	2,500
Total Fat	Less than	65g	80g
Sat Fat	Less than	20g	25g
Cholesterol	Less than	300mg	300mg
Sodium	Less than	2,400mg	2,400mg
Total Carbohydrate		300mg	375mg
Dietary Fiber		25g	30g

Calories per gram:
Fat 9   ●   Carbohydrate 4   ●   Protein 4

How do you compare foods?

Nutritional information can help you to decide whether a food has a little or a lot of something. The table below shows guidelines for determining this. When you look at a food label, get into the habit of thinking about how often and how much of that food you would normally eat. A food may be high in fat and/or sugar, but if you only eat small amounts of it occasionally, then that's okay. For these foods use a "per 100 g" value to see if they contain a little or a lot. This "per 100 g" value is also useful for comparing two similar products, such as sauces, to see which is healthier.

For foods that you eat frequently or in large amounts, it's more appropriate to use the nutrition information given "per serving." Pick a couple of new foods each week and read the labels so you gradually become aware of suitable convenience foods—there's no need to do all of these at once.

How to tell if a food contains a little or a lot of a particular ingredient

A lot	A little
10 grams of sugars	2 grams of sugars
20 grams of fat	3 grams of fat
5 grams of saturated fat	1 grams of saturated fat
3 grams of fiber	0.5 grams of fiber
0.5 grams of sodium	0.1 grams of sodium
1.5 grams of salt	0.3 grams of salt

Summary

- It's okay to eat convenience foods, just follow the guidelines.
- Use our shopping list to select foods that dovetail with your Simple GI Diet.
- A food may be high in fat or sugar, but small, occasional servings are okay!

HEALTHY FOOD TRACKER

This is a tracking system to see how well you're balancing the foods you eat and your lifestyle choices. The highlighted numbers are your targets. You might like to photocopy these pages. Then you can see at a glance how well you're doing at staying with healthy low-GI guidelines.

Which day is it?

Monday
Tuesday
Wednesday
Thursday
Friday
Saturday
Sunday

How are you doing?

Circle the number of portions (servings) you had today of the following:

Starchy carbs—such as bread, cereals, rice, pasta, **potatoes** (choose one serving at each meal).

1 2 (3) 4 5 6 7 8 9 10

Protein foods—such as meat, fish, eggs, cheese, nuts **(once a day only), beans** (only one serving at each meal, max 3 per day).

1 2 (3) 4 5 6 7 8 9 10

Fruit and vegetables (at least 5 a day).

1   2   3   4   (5)   6   7   8   9   10

Sugar-laden and fatty foods (such as cookies, crackers, cakes, pastries, spreads, oils — keep 'em low).

1   2   3   4   5   6   7   8   9   10

Glasses of water (6–8 glasses: 48 to 64 ounces a day).

1   2   3   4   5   6   7   (8)   9   10

Physical activity, such as a brisk walk or running (two 10-minute bursts daily).

1   (2)   3   4   5   6   7   8   9   10

Rank how positive or negative you feel today (5 being the most positive and 1 being the most negative).

1   2   3   4   5

Rank your hunger today (1 means you're starving, 5 means you could do without your next snack).

1   2   3   4   5

Rank your energy today (1 is low, 5 is high).

1   2   3   4   5

Rank your mood today (1 is grumpy, 5 is happy).

1   2   3   4   5

Rank your self-esteem today (1 is the bottom, 5 the top).

1   2   3   4   5

How was breakfast?

☐ Skipped it.

☐ Grab and go, ditched the rules.

☐ Bent the rules but feel okay about it.

☐ Did just what I was supposed to do.

How was lunch?

☐ Skipped it.

☐ Grab and go, ditched the rules.

☐ Bent the rules but feel okay about it.

☐ Did just what I was supposed to do.

How was dinner?

☐ Skipped it.

☐ Grab and go, ditched the rules.

☐ Bent the rules but feel okay about it.

☐ Did just what I was supposed to do.

What about snacks?

☐ Skipped 'em.

☐ Grab and go, ditched the rules.

☐ Bent the rules but feel okay about it.

☐ Did just what I was supposed to do.

How do you rate yourself in general today?

1   2   3   4   5

What do you need right now to make this even better?

How can you achieve this?

What will you do?

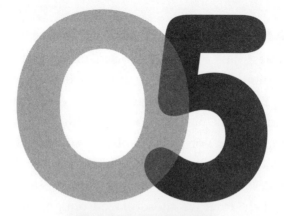

QUICK
AND TASTY
MEAL AND MENU IDEAS

There's no such thing as a free lunch or dinner!

Eating the Simple GI Diet way is like choosing from a Chinese menu—you go for those foods that tempt the taste buds and fit the budget. With GIS eating, you choose a range of tasty treats and make them fit into your daily allowance. You'll find that the more you practice GIS eating, the easier it gets. Remember to picture your plate: veggie, veggie, protein, carbs (Simple GI Diet Rule 4, page 37).

Fill up with a low-GI breakfast

Breakfast, just as grandma used to say, is the most important meal of the day. It *breaks* the *fast* of nighttime. It gets your blood glucose up, which leads to a raised level of blood sugar circulating around your brain, helping you to concentrate. And as you know, low-GIS cereals help stabilize blood glucose, keeping you alert for that mid-morning meeting—and you're less likely to crave those glazed doughnuts. If you can't face a bowl of cereal, try tea and wholegrain toast, a yogurt smoothie, or some unsweetened fruit juice and a few dried apricots.

Always make time for something at breakfast, even if it is something you grab as you speed out of the door. Think especially about your carbohydrate choices: below are some ideas. Turn also to page 83 for the GIS values of our breakfast combos.

Choosing your breakfast carbs

Breakfast cereals: Avoid breakfast cereals with a high sugar content. When choosing cereals look for high-fiber cereals such as All Bran. Muesli is a good choice too. And for a change, add some of your favorite fruits, a sprinkling of chopped walnuts and natural yogurt.

Oatmeal: This is one of the best low-GI breakfast foods ever invented. Instant oatmeal is a convenient substitute, but it is higher in GI since it's more processed.

Top Tip: Try making some speedy oatmeal in the microwave. Check the package for instructions.

Bread: Toast is always a favorite but choose your bread carefully. Go for grainy varieties such as flaxseed or multigrain. For variety, why not try toasted raisin bread.

Milk and juices: If you've run out the door without even thinking about food, you could pick up a drink-able yogurt or an individual carton of milk on your way to work. Look for low-fat milkshakes and smoothies.

Fill up with a low-GI lunch

Your low-GI breakfast and mid-morning snack will keep your energy levels raised throughout the morning. That mid-morning snack not only keeps blood glucose stable, it also prevents you from overeating at lunchtime. And the effect of a low GI breakfast and mid-morning snack will last til lunchtime. By then, it's time to refuel with a "right carbs" lunch.

● Make or buy sandwiches made with suitable bread and low-fat fillings such as lean meat, chicken or

Top Tip: Got time? Why not make a smoothie—blend together your favorite fruit (fresh or canned in juice) with skim or 2% milk and nonfat yogurt.

fish, and use plenty of lettuce. Avoid mayonnaise, since it is high in fat. Instead, choose mustard, pickles, chutney, salsa or lemon juice to add flavor.

● Create your own salad using a variety of salad vegetables, adding canned mixed beans (count as 2 GISs), tuna (1 GIS), mozzarella cheese (3 GISs) or egg (2 GISs). Avoid oil-based salad dressings. For a real zing, why not try hot sauce, lemon juice and black pepper?

● Make your own pasta salad: boil your favorite pasta, add some chopped ham, tuna or reduced-fat cheese. Toss in some extra beans and salad

Eat these...	Instead of ...
Muesli, oatmeal, bran cereals	Cornflakes, puffed wheat
Grainy bread, such as soft-grain white or multigrain	White or whole wheat bread
Unsweetened fruit juice, diet drinks or water	Sugared soft drinks
Boiled new potatoes in their skin, or sweet potatoes	Mashed potatoes or French fries
Lean meat, poultry without the skin, fish	Fatty meat
Small muffins	Danish pastry or doughnut
Lentil-based dishes	Meat-based dishes
Oatmeal cookies	Wheat-based cookies

vegetables and mix together with low-fat natural yogurt and herbs for a creamy dressing.

● Turn to page 86 for the GIS values of our lunch combos.

Choosing your lunch and main-meal carbs

Bread: Choose grainy, dense breads with whole seeds for your sandwiches or with your main meal. Multigrain, flaxseed, rye, 100 percent stoneground whole wheat, oatbran and barley breads are all good choices.

Potatoes: Most potatoes have a high GI, new potatoes are slightly lower. They are, however, a nutritious part of the diet, so rather than cutting them out altogether make sure you include other low-GI carbohydrates with them. Alternatively, why not try sweet potatoes, which have a low GI and taste delicious when baked or microwaved.

Pasta: Enjoy with your lunch-time salad or as your main meal. Most pasta has a low GI. Cook until *al dente* and remember, watch what you serve pasta with — avoid creamy high-calorie sauces.

Rice: Choose basmati rice, long-grain or brown rice. For an alternative to pasta or rice, bulgur wheat (cracked wheat) has a low GI and tastes great in salads.

Beans, lentils and peas: As well as being low-GI foods, these legumes are a great source of protein, iron and

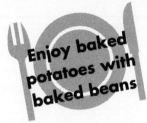

Enjoy baked potatoes with baked beans

fiber. Include them in your meals whenever possible—have stir-fried beans, beany casseroles and soups, or just toss them into any salad; they will help lower the GI of the meal.

Vegetables, fruit and salad: Great for lowering the GI of a meal and full of important antioxidant vitamins and minerals. Vegetables, fruit and salad should always appear in your lunch-time and main meals. Fresh, frozen and canned fruit and vegetables all count toward your five-a-day recommended intake—the more variety and color the better.

Dinner time!

Having a dinner dilemma? Want something quick and easy to prepare after a hard day at work? Or do you want to impress friends or family but still stick to your low-Simple GI Diet? There are four important points to consider to ensure your meal is healthy and well balanced:

- Base your meal on a low-GI carbohydrate—pasta,

noodles, sweet potato, grains such as bulgur wheat or barley, basmati rice, new potatoes, beans, peas and lentils.

- Make sure you include generous amounts of vegetables or salad, or ideally both!
- Always include some protein such as lean meat, poultry, fish, eggs, reduced-fat cheese, legumes, or a handful of nuts. You could use peas, beans, lentils and chickpeas to extend meat dishes. For example, mixing some lentils with a bolognese sauce can make it go further, while lowering the GI.
- Watch the fat. Use healthy cooking methods that require little oil, such as stir-frying, steaming, poaching and baking. Avoid high-fat sauces and dressings that contain butter, cream or lots of oil. Look for reduced-fat dairy products such as low-

Save a GIS or two

Eat this ...	Instead of ...	Save ...
Oatcakes	Rice cakes	3.5 GISs
Raisin Bread	Waffle	2.5 GISs
Drinkable yogurt	Fresh cranberry juice	2 GISs
Tortillas	White bread	2.5 GISs
Pita bread	Baguette	4 GISs
Canned pears	Canned peaches	1 GIS
Dried figs	Dried dates	1 GIS
Basmati rice	Jasmine rice	5 GISs
New potatoes	French fries	3 GISs

fat yogurt or reduced-fat crème fraîche or cheese.

For healthy low-carb dinner combos, turn to page 89.

In a jiffy

The same rules apply if you are eating a prepared meal. When choosing a packaged meal make sure it contains some low-GI carbohydrate and some lean protein ingredients.

Many supermarkets now offer a healthier low-fat range, which can be a good option. These may contain very few vegetables so always add extra or serve with a side salad. And if you don't have a clue to the GIS value of a meal, simply choose the types of foods that you know are low-GI and add some GIS-free goodies.

Desserts

Fortunately many desserts are based on fruit and dairy products, both having a low GI. Fruit cocktail with low-fat ice cream has 3.5 GISs and a carton of diet yogurt offers one virtuous GIS.

Vegetarian-style eating

Many vegetarian foods have a low GI. It's the way you cook them and what you mix with them that counts:

● Keep your foods as whole as possible.

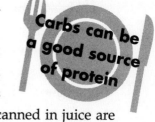

Carbs can be a good source of protein

- Remember that beans and lentils are especially low-GI foods.
- Many fruits also have a low GI. Examples are apples, cherries, grapefruit, pears, strawberries and plums. Peaches and pears canned in juice are also great choices.
- Red lentils, haricot beans, French beans and runner beans have an exceptionally low GI.
- Go easy on the cheese. It contains around 30 percent fat, mostly saturated. Grate it to go further or choose reduced-fat versions.
- Don't be fooled into thinking that all foods bought from a health food store are good for you. Many can be high in fat and sugar, and even though they may be made with whole wheat flour, they are not necessarily healthy.
- Bangladeshi rice is the lowest-GI rice.

A leaf from the olive tree

The Mediterranean way of eating, with an abundance of olive oil, fish, nuts, fruit and veggies, has been associated with a lower risk of conditions such as coronary heart disease and cancer. Interestingly, the total amount of fat eaten by people who live in Mediterranean countries is actually quite high. But take a closer look and you'll see that it's high in monounsaturated fats (such as olive oil) and omega-3 fats (such as those found in oily fish). Studies on "Med-eating" support the idea that opting for the right types of fat may be more important than getting your fat intake really low.

Research suggests that as little as one ounce of oily fish a day can significantly lower the incidence of heart disease. People in Mediterranean countries also have a much higher intake of fruit and vegetables, so they benefit from a good antioxidant intake. They eat more garlic, and this characteristic ingredient of Mediterranean cuisine also has therapeutic properties. Garlic has been shown to thin the blood, helping it to flow more smoothly. Garlic also contains the natural antibiotic allicin.

Study after study has shown that nuts such as walnuts, almonds and peanuts, commonly consumed in the Mediterranean countries, are beneficial to health. Rich in monounsaturated fats, they are, however, high in calories, so keep to a small handful (about one ounce) a day, especially if you're watching your waistline.

Taking a leaf from the olive tree, it makes sense to incorporate the healthy aspects of Mediterranean cuisine into a balanced diet. So, enjoy the Mediterranean musts—garlic, fruit and vegetables, fish, a glass of red wine, beans and lentils, a handful of nuts. Remember, too, to eat slowly, savor your food and linger over your meal.

Meal Combos

These "Combos" contain calculated meal choices for breakfast, lunch and dinner. You can swap them around on different days. They are your choices for lazy days, when you don't want to think too much about what to eat. You can also plan your shopping around them. In fact, there are seven or more different combos for each meal occasion so you can just do one big trip to the grocery store and you're set for a week.

Pick and choose from this buffet of delights—opt for the meals that fit in with your GISs. You'll soon know which ones are your regular "must-haves." For in-between-meal goodies, choose from the snacks below or refer to Snack Attack (Chapter 6).

Remember Simple GI Diet Rule 1—*Eat three meals and three snacks every day.*

These combos are filling and balanced meal choices. If you're looking for a meal with lower GISs, feel free to leave out some items, or have them later as one of your snacks.

Combo Breakfast Choices	GISs
1 All Bran (5 tbsp) and	2
2% milk (7 oz)	
1 small banana	2
	4
2 Branflakes (4 tbsp) and	4
2% milk (7 oz)	
1 fresh apple	0.5
	4.5
3 Oatmeal (6 tbsp), made	3.5
2% milk (3 oz) and water (as needed)	
Honey (1 tsp)	1
Tomato juice (5 oz)	0
	4.5
4 Muesli (3 tbsp) and 2%	4
2% milk (7 oz)	
Pineapple juice,	1.5
unsweetened (5 oz)	
	5.5
5 Special K (5 tbsp) and	4
2% milk (7 oz)	
1 fresh grapefruit	0
	4

Combo Breakfast Choices	GISs
6 Bran Flakes (4 tbsp) and 2% milk (7 oz)	4
Poached eggs (2)	1.5
	5.5
7 Instant hot oatmeal made with 2% milk (7 oz)	4.5
1 fresh pear	0.5
	5
8 Peanut butter (2 tsp) on 1 slice of whole wheat bread	3.5
Cantaloupe melon (½)	2
	5.5
9 Whole wheat bread (2 slices) with low-fat spread and banana (1)	**6**
10 Multigrain bread (2 slices) with scrambled eggs (2) and tomato	**6**
11 Whole wheat bread (2 slices) with butter (1 tsp) and poached eggs (2)	**8**

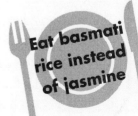

Eat basmati rice instead of jasmine

Combo Lunch Choices with Dessert	GISs
1 Multigrain bread (2 slices) with low-fat spread (1 tsp), tuna (small can) and cucumber	4
Reduced-fat chocolate pudding (about 5 oz)	1.5
	5.5
2 Wheat tortilla (1) with chicken (3 slices) and mixed green salad	4
Yogurt, low-fat or non-fat (5 oz)	1
	5
3 Wheat tortilla (1) with mozzarella cheese (small matchbox-size piece, chopped), tomato and basil	4.5
Grapes (15)	2
	6.5
4 Multigrain bread (2 slices), low-fat spread (1 tsp), ham (2 medium-size slices) and salad	5
Olives (10)	0.5
	5.5
5 Multigrain bread (2 slices) with low-fat spread (1 tsp), mozzarella cheese (1 slice), fresh basil and tomato	5.5
Apple (1)	0.5
	6

Combo Lunch Choices with Dessert	GISs
6 Pumpernickel bread (2 slices) and low-fat spread (1 tsp), ham (2 slices), mixed green salad	5.5
Chocolate flavored 2% milk (7 oz)	1
	6.5
7 Baked potato with low-fat spread (1 tsp), cottage cheese (about 4.5 oz) and sliced bell peppers	6.5
Plums (3)	0.5
	7
8 Whole wheat bread (2 slices) with low-fat spread (1 tsp), cottage cheese (small tub) and shredded cucumber and lettuce	6.5
Reduced-fat chocolate pudding	1.5
	8
9 Baked potato with low-fat spread (1 tsp), tuna (small can) and corn (3 tbsp)	7
Packet minestrone soup	0
	7

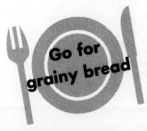

Go for grainy bread

Combo Lunch Choices with Dessert	GISs
10 Whole wheat bread (2 slices) with low-fat spread (1 tsp), feta and tomato	7
Canned peaches, in juices (6 slices) with sugar-free Jell-O	0.5
	7.5
11 Baked potato with low-fat spread (1 tsp), half-fat cheddar cheese (3 tbsp grated) and side salad (fat-free dressing)	9.5
Fresh strawberries (5 oz)	0
	9.5
12 Baguette (1 small) with low-fat spread (1 tsp), shrimp (small jar, about 3.5 oz) and mixed green salad (fat-free dressing)	10.5
Fresh pear	0.5
	11

Main Meal Choices	GISs

(Recipes and portion sizes for all of these meals are in Chapter 8.)

1 Garlic Mushrooms	0
Cod Kebabs with Fresh Dill	1.5
Mixed salad	0
Tortilla wrap	3
	4.5

Main Meal Choices	GISs
2 Turkey Stroganoff	1.5
Basmati rice (6 tbsp)	2.5
Grilled tomato salad	0
Orange juice, unsweetened (5 oz)	1.5
	5.5
3 Haddock with Thai Green Pepper and Basil Sauce	2.5
Instant noodles (5 tbsp)	2
Side salad in fat-free dressing	0
Jell-O with whole strawberries	0
	4.5
4 Salmon Steaks in Garlicky Balsamic Vinegar	3.5
Boiled egg fettucine (5 tbsp)	1.5
Steamed asparagus tips	0
Peaches, canned in juice (6 slices)	0.5
	5.5
5 Couscous with Peppers and Red Onion	4.5
Chili beans (7 oz)	1
Lettuce, cucumber, tomato, red onion salad	0
	5.5

Main Meal Choices	GISs
6 Yellow Squash and Leek Soup	0
Mediterranean Pasta	5
Green herby salad (watercress, mixed lettuce leaves, fresh herbs, lime juice, black pepper)	0
Low-fat natural yogurt	1
Fresh cherries (12)	0.5
	6.5
7 Beef Chow Mein	7
Stir-fried Baby Corn	0
Tomato juice (5 oz)	0
	7

Starters and Sides*

(See Chapter 8 for recipes and portion sizes. If GISs are 0, eat as much as you want!)

	GISs
Al Dente Asparagus	0
Balsamic French Beans	0
Beef Tomatoes with Black Olives	1
Cabbage with Fennel Seeds	0
Chili and Honey Chicken Wings	2
Chili and Lime Arugula Leaves	0
Chili Peanut Popcorn	2.5
Cucumber and Mint Cooler	0

Curried Okra	0
Garlic Mushrooms	0
Gherkin and Onion Pickle	0
Grilled Tomato Salad	0
Herby Baby Spinach and Beansprouts	0
Roasted Vegetables	0
Jell-O with Whole Strawberries	0
Savoy Cabbage with Caraway Seeds	0
Speedy Salsa Sauce	0
Spiced Vegetables	0
Stir-fried Babycorn	0
Wheat-free Tabouleh	0
Yellow Squash and Leek Soup	0
Zucchini Boats	0

* these dishes can also be used as snacks

Grab-a-snack	GISs
Chewy granola and dried fruit bar (45–50 g)	4.5
Crunchy granola and dried fruit bar (45–50 g)	4.5

Nuts*:	
Almonds (10–12)	3
Cashews (15)	3.5
Peanuts, dry roasted (1 oz)	3
Peanuts, roasted and salted (1 oz)	3
Walnuts (6 halves)	3

* strictly once a day

Grab-a-snack	GISs
Popcorn, plain, popped (5 tbsp)	4
Soup:	
Minestrone, dried (1 bowl)	0
Tomato, dried (1 bowl)	0.5
Yogurt:	
Non-fat (5 oz)	1
Low-fat, natural (5 oz)	1

Sample menus

Below are five sample menu plans from people who've followed the Simple GI Diet. The 17- and 20-GIS plans are from women, and the 22- and 25-GIS plans are from men. There's also a vegetarian one that you can enjoy if this is your preference. These quick and easy menus will inspire you with many more ideas and show you it's simple to put the diet into practice. You might like to jot down your own plans so that you can reuse them to save you time. For portion sizes check the GIS tables at the back of the book.

17-GIS sample menu, Start-it Phase

Breakfast:	All Bran with 2% milk	2.5
	Fresh pear	0.5

Snack:	Chewy granola bar	4.5
Lunch:	Garlic and tomato herb fettucine	
	(request no oil when dining out)	
	5 tablespoons fettucine	1.5
	Tomatoes, onions, herbs, garlic	0
	Mixed free salad, no dressing	0
Snack:	Apple	0.5
Dinner:	Spiced lemon sole with potatoes and vegetables	
	Lemon sole, grilled	1
	Broccoli, steamed	0
	Baby corn	0
	Carrots, 6 tablespoons	1
	Potatoes, boiled	3
	Chili sauce, salt/pepper	0
Fruit:	8 prunes	1.5
Night snack:	Low- or non-fat yogurt	1
Unlimited still water		0
Total		**17**

Additional free daily allowance:
7 ounces 2% milk 0.5

20-GIS sample menu, Lose-it Phase

Breakfast:	Reduced-sugar muesli with 2% milk	4
Snack:	Fun-size Snickers® bar	2
Lunch:	Home-made weekend veggie rice	
	Basmati rice	2.5

	Kidney beans (canned)	2
	Tomatoes (canned)	0
	Onions, herbs and spices	0
Snack:	Low-fat natural yogurt	1
Dinner:	Chili chicken with sweet potato and salad	
	Chicken breast	2
	Baked sweet potato	3
	Broccoli, steamed	0
	Chili sauce	0
	Large side salad (celery, tomato, cucumber, lettuce, red onion)	0
Night snack:	Peanut butter on a slice of whole wheat toast	3.5
Unlimited still water		0
Total		**20**

Additional free daily allowance:
        7 ounces 2% milk 0.5

22-GIS sample menu, Start-it Phase

Breakfast:	Oatmeal, made with milk and water	3.5
	Tomato juice with Worcester sauce	0
Snack:	Banana	2
Lunch:	Multigrain bread (toasted)	3.5
	Baked beans, canned in tomato sauce	2
Snack:	15 grapes	2
Dinner:	Roast chicken with new potatoes,	

	carrots, peas and gravy	
	3 slices roast chicken	2
	4 boiled new potatoes	3
	3 tablespoons peas	2
	GIS-free stir-fried baby corn	0
	Instant gravy	0.5
Snack:	Reduced-fat chocolate pudding	1.5
Total		**22**

Additional free daily allowance:

7 ounces 2% milk 0.5

½ pint (about 9.5 ounces) of beer from alcohol allowance

25-GIS sample menu, Lose-it Phase

Breakfast:	Shredded wheat and 2% milk	4.5
Snack:	10 almonds	3
Lunch:	Lentil soup	2
	Multigrain bread, 2 slices	3.5
Snack:	Orange	1.5
Dinner:	Grilled steak with fries, mushrooms and side salad	
	5 oz rump steak, lean, grilled	2
	Fries, 6 tablespoons 5 percent fat, frozen, oven baked	5
	Mushrooms, stir-fried in a little oil	2
	Mixed "free" salad vegetables	0
Snack:	Pears, canned in juice	1.5

Total		**25**

Additional free daily allowance:
7 ounces 2% milk 0.5

25-GIS sample menu, vegetarian

Breakfast:	2 slices barley bread	3
	Low-fat spread, scraping	0.5
	1 banana, sliced	2
Snack:	3 plums	0.5
	1 pear	0.5
Lunch:	2 slices white bread	5.5
	Low-fat spread, scraping	0.5
	1 oz feta cheese 2.5	
	Tomato	0
	1 apple	0.5
Snack:	6 walnut halves	3
Dinner:	Lentil and vegetable casserole	
	(Lentils, cupful of cooked [2 oz raw dried] baked in oven with mixed vegetables, canned tomatoes and vegetable stock)	1
	Brown rice, 6 tablespoons	2.5
	1 nonfat yogurt	1
Snack:	½ cantaloupe	2
Total		**25**

Additional free daily allowance:
7 ounces 2% milk 0.5

Summary

- Link pleasure to your meal and menu planning and reach your happy weight in a safe and sustainable way.
- See your plate with two vegetable portions (v, v), plus one protein (p) and low-GI carb (c): veggie, veggie, protein, carbs!
- Think of your meal as two veggies plus meat and one carb, and it'll help you keep your portions in perspective.

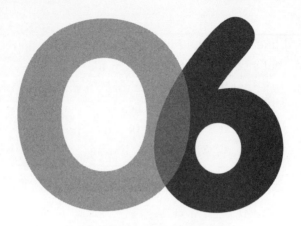

SNACK ATTACK

No time for breakfast ... rushing to work ... quick snack on the way home. Sound familiar? With our hectic lifestyles today, eating on the run is becoming more common, and so keeping an eye on fats and figures can be difficult. What's more, fast snack food isn't necessarily healthy food, and often convenience overrides health. So, how can the Simple GI Diet overcome the snacking blips? What thoughts will influence your choices?

Choices and consequences

When it comes to making a choice, for example, between that glazed doughnut or an apple, which one will you choose? Hmmm—tough choice, eh? Okay, so we all like to indulge from time to time and, on occasion, that's cool. What you might like to think about, though, is that the choices you make today shape your future tomorrow, both physically, in terms of your future health, and mentally, because they affect your overall sense of well-being. Eating that doughnut today can have an effect on your health, your waistline, and how you feel about yourself once the short-term pleasure it gave you is over.

Healthy snacks can be good for you, however. For example, they're helpful in keeping you alert in the middle of the day. With GI eating, snacks can be your best friends because they help to keep your blood sugar levels steady. What's more, they can positively help you watch that waistline, since a feeling of fullness means you're less likely to raid the fridge as soon as you drop your coat in the hallway.

Having a snack attack?

Here's the low-down on some well-known favorites. How do your choices measure up?

Crudités and dips: A crunchy way to get your anti-oxidants. Fill up on the following to reduce the likelihood of overdoing the calories later. Carrot sticks, cucumber, celery and other crudité veggies are low in GISs. Opt for healthy dips such as those based on low-fat yogurt, such as Indian raita or Greek tzatziki, that are high in calcium, or tomatoes, such as salsa, that are high in lycopene.

Spice up your chickpeas: Chickpeas are a great source of fiber and protein. Start with about one cup. Add some fresh lime juice, chili and chopped coriander leaves. Toss them onto a bed of mixed red onion and watercress salad and you have a substantial snack for only 2.5 GISs. (If you boil them from dried, it comes to only 1.5 GISs.)

Peanuts: Nuts can help to fill you up so that you are less likely to overeat. They contain healthy monounsaturated fats and a range of vitamins and minerals. Scientific research suggests that 1 oz of peanuts daily may suppress hunger and so promote weight loss, lower blood cholesterol levels, and reduce the risk of type 2 diabetes in women. There is also extensive research on almonds and walnuts. That's why certain nuts are encouraged in the Simple GI Diet once a day. Unsalted nuts are best.

Rice cakes: These are low in calories, yes, but high in GI. Consequently, rice cakes have a high GIS value. Swap two rice cakes for two oatmeal cookies and you halve the GISs you spend.

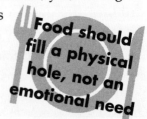

Food should fill a physical hole, not an emotional need

Olives: Satisfying, moist and rich in healthy mono-unsaturated fat. Very low in GISs; keep to recommended portions. Taste not waist!

Popcorn: A healthy snack, high in fiber and protein, but higher in GISs than regular corn, because of the way it changes form when cooked. Make it yourself with a couple of tablespoons of popping corn and a teaspoon of oil, cover and watch 'em pop! Or try Chili Peanut Popcorn (recipe page 131) which lowers the GISs by mixing the corn with peanuts.

Snacks in the office
Here are some handy low GIS carbs that you can take to the office. If a healthy snack is accessible, it'll be easier for you to keep to your GIS rules.

- Drinkable yogurt
- Milkshake powder and skim or 2% milk
- Fresh fruit
- Individual canned fruit in juice
- Dried fruit

Eat ...	Instead of ...
Oatcakes	Rice cakes
Fun-size Snickers® bar	Milk chocolate bar
Half a dozen walnut halves	Pretzels
Olives	Cheese chunks
Tzatziki dip made from low-fat yogurt	Sour cream dip

- Low-fat or non-fat yogurt
- Dried soup

GIS-free snacks

Get creative and conjure up a delectable GIS-free snack in seconds by using our quick and easy recipes (page 140). Here's the low-down:

Garlic Mushrooms

Cabbage with Fennel Seeds

Grilled Tomato Salad

Zucchini Boats

Chili and Lime Arugula Leaves

Yellow Squash and Leek Soup

Savoy Cabbage with Caraway Seeds

Herby Baby Spinach and Beansprouts

Gherkin and Onion Pickle

Stir-fried Baby Corn

Curried Okra

Balsamic French Beans

Roasted Vegetables

Speedy Salsa Sauce

Cucumber and Mint Cooler

Spiced Vegetables

Al Dente Asparagus

Wheat-free Tabouleh

Jell-O with Whole Strawberries

Cook-a-snack

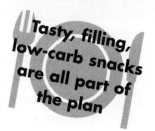

Tasty, filling, low-carb snacks are all part of the plan

Figure out your GISs from the raw ingredients for these substantial snacks or light meals. (Check GIS Tables at the back of the book for portion sizes.)

- Cheat's pizza — take a slice of pita bread, smother it in tomato purée and add lots of veggies, such as green peppers, mushrooms, zucchini and tomatoes. Top with a bit of grated cheese and a few halved olives.

- Boil up some pasta and throw in some canned tuna, fresh basil, garlic and some cubed reduced-fat feta cheese.

- Southern sweet potato fries — peel and cut a sweet potato into French fries or rounds. Boil until just cooked. Drizzle over a little olive oil and flavor with Cajun seasoning, black pepper and a touch of lemon juice. Grill or bake.

- Baked zucchini — cut a zucchini lengthwise and sprinkle with coarse black pepper, balsamic vinegar and some spray oil. Smother with toasted sesame seeds. Bake or microwave.

And a couple of chilled snacks …

- Crudités — chop up your favorite raw veggies and

serve with raita (natural low-fat yogurt mixed with grated cucumber and cumin seeds).

● Banana and peach smoothie—in a blender, whip up some low-fat fruit yogurt with a banana and some drained canned peaches.

Don't dehydrate

Did you know that around 60 percent of your body weight is water? We continually need to replace the amount we lose each day in our breath, sweat and urine. You need even more fluid if you're in a centrally heated or air-conditioned environment.

Drink at least 48 to 64 ounces of fluid each day. Some people find that keeping a bottle of water on their desk makes this easier, especially since seeing water may make you more conscious of your thirst. However, you needn't restrict yourself to plain water. Have a variety of drinks, such as unsweetened fruit juice, sugar-free soft drinks, low-fat milk and flavored waters. You may have a few cups of tea and coffee, too, if you like.

Many soft drinks and fruit juices contain sugar and

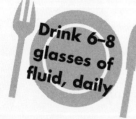
Drink 6-8 glasses of fluid, daily

this raises their Glycemic Index. So drinking large amounts of fruit juice, even if unsweetened, may make your blood glucose rise sharply. This is because sugar in liquid form is rapidly absorbed by the body. If you like fresh fruit juice, drink it with a meal rather than on its own. Tomato juice is particularly low in GISs, so choose it in preference to higher-GIS sweetened drinks. Be particularly cautious with high-energy glucose drinks—they send your blood glucose up very quickly and therefore are higher in GISs.

An easy way to check if you're drinking enough is to look at the color of your urine the next time you go to the bathroom. If it's pale and there's lots of it, then you're probably drinking enough. If you're passing less urine and it's darker, then this could be a sign of dehydration.

The comfort cushion

The key to long-term good snacking is to have a healthy relationship with all types of food. Food has emotional, psychological and social aspects to it, so it pays to examine your attitude towards food. Aim to get the right balance most of the time. As soon as you say to yourself that you must avoid a food, what happens? That food becomes even more desirable. Challenge your thinking and attitudes towards food.

Get into the habit of knowing which are the low-GIS foods and opt for these, often. And remember that high-GIS foods aren't *bad* foods—there's a place for all kinds of food. You will soon find that you automatically know which of your daily foods are lower and which are a little higher in GISs. With this knowledge, you can include a healthy mix of foods with confidence.

The GIS IQ Test

Question:

Are you a snack-o-holic? If so, when are you likely to indulge?

Choice 1: I go for snacks when I feel hungry, but it's usually fruit, some veggies I keep in the fridge, a granola bar or a few cashews.

Great! You are conscious of when you're eating, and you are making healthy choices.

Choice 2: When I'm on the go, I'll attack the closest convenience store and look for a sugar fix.

Your blood sugar is more likely to fluctuate from high to low if you graze on sweet stuff. Not such a good idea.

Choice 3: When I'm feeling down in the dumps, or a bit under the weather, I could eat all day …

Consequently, your meals and snacks may be less regular, which may lead you to make unhealthy food choices. You may be more likely to pile on the pounds since you're less conscious of what you're eating.

Results:

Choice 1: You'll appreciate the high energy and an overall feel-good state, which also means the likelihood of a positive frame of mind.

Choice 2: Choose more filling options like a light wholegrain sandwich, a small packet of nuts or a banana. Give yourself an extra boost of motivation and think about the end goal—what it is that you really want, and direct your thoughts in that direction!

Choice 3: Today's choices become tomorrow's consequences and that includes how you are choosing to feel. Think about supporting someone else, in some small way. This way, you'll relieve yourself of the burden of self-obsession! By focusing on others, you'll feel uplifted and are therefore more likely to get back on track with your own goals.

Summary

● Snacks can be good for your mental performance and they help keep blood glucose levels steady. With GIS eating, low-GI snacks can be your best friends.

● Keep a daily food and mood diary so you can see what makes you over-indulge (see page 50).

● Get into the habit of knowing the low-GIS snacks—maybe keep them handy at work and make them a regular item on your shopping list.

● Distract yourself. Make a creative and fun list of all the things that would work for you.

● Treat your new healthy food choices as a fresh way of life. If you lapse occasionally, just acknowledge it and start again.

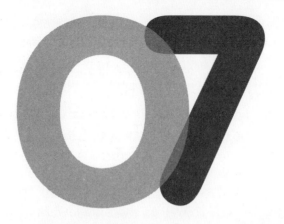

EATING OUT THE SIMPLE GI DIET WAY

Your body is a temple ...

And sometimes it's a nightclub! A little of what you like does you good, but too much can bring about a different set of consequences, including weight gain.

Eating out is one of the pleasures of life, and when you're dieting, there's no reason why you can't join in the fun. Whether it's a business meeting over lunch, dinner with friends or family, or fast-food take-out

Ultimately your actions are driven by your deepest desire or intention.

when you're on the move, eating out is a part of our lives that's here to stay. And it can be part of your new healthier Simple GI Diet lifestyle.

Pain versus pleasure

Even if you don't know the GIS value of your indulgence, by following our simple tips you can make healthy choices, as well as choosing lower-GI options. More and more restaurants and fast-food outlets are taking notice of the increasing demand for healthier menus. Remember, in a restaurant *you* are the customer and can request changes in the way food is cooked and served. Simply ask. You're paying for it! Here are some tips on eating out to help you on your way.

For starters, no need to advertise that you're "on a diet." Your friends will probably start saying, "Oh, you can just have one today," and you might give in to temptation. Instead, hold your head up high and order these delicious choices with confidence, since GIS-eating isn't about dieting, it's about balance. When you don't tell yourself you're "on a diet," the rest of the gang will want to know the secrets of your successful weight loss.

Avoid going to a restaurant ravenous for the next mouthful. Instead, grab a piece of fruit or GIS-free food on the way. Another tip: Get into the habit of putting your fork and knife down after every mouthful. It's amazing how much longer your meal will last.

Remember that you're there to enjoy yourself, so long as this isn't something you do five days a week! Make a mental note of what you've chosen so you can keep track of your GISs and make up for it at other times if you have overdone it.

Feedback is the currency of life

Your body is the best feedback mechanism available. There will be negative feelings that you link to when you overeat, have one drink too many, or smoke too much. Remember how your head feels? How your mouth resembles the bottom of a parrot's cage? Or the effects on your digestive system of that spicy curry? You might have felt bloated, had a distended stomach, or needed to slouch in the armchair with no energy, nursing the mother of all hang- 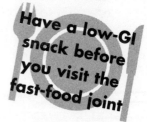 overs, with the words "Never again!" ringing in your ears.

As you sit in a restaurant or get in line for a burger, think about these feelings so that you'll start making wise choices. Link more and more pleasurable feelings to your new choices, knowing that they are taking you nearer to the "new" you. Think about your increased energy levels, the boost in confidence and self-esteem you are getting, and all the other benefits

Have a low-GI snack before you visit the fast-food joint

of getting nearer to that ideal, happy weight. Next time you're eating out, perhaps you'll be in the much-dreamt-about little black dress!

In the restaurant ...

This very week, when you've finally made the decision to start your new healthy living plan, guess what? You're inundated with dinner and party offers! This will test just how committed you really are. Get through this and you've shown what you're made of. No need to join the "Lonely Hearts" club! The first step is to overcome your habit of ordering the richest, most indulgent food on the menu. You'll need some focus and determination to succeed — but succeed you can.

All patterns can be broken. Anything learned can be unlearned. Enjoy and continue to draw on the essential tools offered in this book to support you in making the life that you really want. Tell yourself "I always choose healthily" and look for ways to support this. Here's how you can begin to make those changes by choosing wisely when you're eating out.

Eating Italian

Italian food is not just pizza and pasta: many menus feature grilled meats, chicken and seafood dishes served with plenty of fresh vegetables, all of which can be healthier choices. Here are some GIS tips:

- Most pasta has a low GI, but the sauces served with it can be laden with fat and calories. Order pasta with a fresh tomato sauce, which tends to be lower in fat than cream-based sauces, and say "no" to the Parmesan cheese. Ask for your plate to be half filled with a crunchy selection of mixed salad leaves and the other half filled with the pasta of your choice.

- Go for a thin-crust pizza with lots of low-GI vegetable toppings. Steer clear of extra cheese and processed pepperoni.

- Ask for a GIS-free salad with your meal. For the dressing, opt for balsamic vinegar or a squeeze of lemon juice and a sprinkling of herbs.

- If you are having a grilled meat or chicken dish, ask for the sauce on the side so you have control over how much you eat, or go without. Ask for unbuttered vegetables and boiled new potatoes in their skins (4 GISs). Don't be tempted to have the French fries since these have a higher GI and are high in fat (6 GISs).

- Remember, you may be starving when you're waiting for your meal to arrive but those bread GISs still count. Rather than garlic bread, choose a healthier low-GI starter such as chunky vegetable soup, melon, Mozzarella and tomato salad or tuna salad with an oil-free dressing.

Eating Indian

If you're ordering group dishes, be careful how much you eat. This is a common pitfall in Indian, Chinese and Thai restaurants. Give yourself a full plate at the beginning of a meal, eat slowly and stop when you've finished. Indian cuisine can be GIS-friendly. Just avoid the high-fat fried foods and heavy, butter-based sauces.

● For the main course, go for a dahl dish, which is made from lentils. There are many different types to choose from. Ask the waiter which dahls are less puréed and choose those — they have a lower Glycemic Index. For calculating your GISs, use the cooked dahl value (a cupful has only 3.5 GISs).

● Opt for chicken, shrimp or vegetable dishes, rather than lamb or beef, which tend to be higher in fat. You might see a layer of orange oil on the top — scoop your serving from underneath.

● Go for tandoori chicken or chicken tikka as they are cooked quickly without added fat. Choose plain boiled rice, and cucumber and mint raita, a cooling low-GI accompaniment.

● Avoid the richer dishes such as korma, pasanda, masala, and deep-fried samosas and bhajis. Save your GISs for bigger portions of better choices.

● Accompany your meal with some steamed or boiled basmati rice, and stay away from pilau and biryanis, unless you only have a small amount.

- Add a GIS-free salad to whatever you're having. In Indian restaurants, they're usually dressed in lime or lemon juice and these acids can help lower the GI of the meal.
- Ask for your popadums to be grilled or microwaved—they taste just as crunchy as fried ones, and have less than half the fat. You might start a trend. Some restaurants now serve this routinely.
- Finish with a fresh fruit salad.

Remember Simple GI Diet Rule 5: *Have at least one low-GIS food at each meal and always have a snack.*

Eating Chinese

A Chinese menu will feature plenty of vegetables, rice and noodles with lots of low-GI, low-fat dishes to choose from. Using chopsticks makes you eat more slowly, so you could end up using fewer GISs!

- Choose healthy starters such as soups and satay dishes with chili dipping sauces. Avoid deep-fried foods like spring rolls.
- Opt for anything on the menu that is steamed, such as whole steamed fish with ginger, steamed vegetables and steamed rice.
- Stir-fried dishes are a great choice, as this method of cooking uses very little oil. Select dishes with added vegetables to keep your GISs low.

- Jasmine rice is high in GISs (a whopping 8 GISs), as is Asian-style sticky rice (7 GISs). Choose steamed rice rather than special fried varieties. You would be better off with noodles (egg, rice or mung bean—allow 3 GISs) as a lower-GI alternative.

- For dessert finish with fresh fruit or some canned lychees (leave the syrup).

Eating Thai

Thai dishes can be very healthy. They typically include small amounts of meat, seafood or tofu with vegetables and spicy sauce. Most are good choices. Follow the advice for Chinese food above. Also …

- Avoid the deep-fried starters and go for clear soups, chicken satay or steamed vegetable dumplings, which are lower in fat yet high in taste.

- Thai curries contain coconut milk, which is high in saturated fat. Instead, choose stir-fries or noodle dishes—add some extra chili sauce if you dare!

Eating French

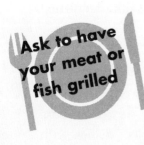

Ask to have your meat or fish grilled

French restaurants serve many dishes that are generally drenched in rich creamy sauces, but there will always be something on the menu that is healthy or can be made healthier.

- For starters, dig into a plate of crudités, and choose low-fat dressings or healthy dips based on tomato or yogurt. Vegetable soup can be a healthy lower-GI option, but avoid the creamy ones. Remember that the puréed soups will be higher in GI than the more chunky ones. If you're eating bread, select whole-grain breads or rolls. Ask for a melon or shrimp cocktail dressed in lime juice.

- Ask to have your meat or fish grilled without oil, or just a small amount. Avoid the creamy, butter-rich sauces and ask for some fresh lemon wedges or French mustard instead. If you have been given sauce, put it aside before you dig in.

- Choose unbuttered new potatoes with your meal rather than mashed potatoes, baked potatoes or French fries. New potatoes have a lower GI. Or go for noodles or couscous instead. Make sure you have lots of unbuttered vegetables or salad.

- If you're tempted by the dessert menu, make a beeline for sweets with fruit and plain ice cream. Remember, they may still be huge portions, so ask for two spoons and share it with your dinner companion.

Eating Mexican

Many of the food choices at Mexican restaurants can be high GI and are often fried or served with creamy sauces, so choose carefully.

- Mexican tortilla wraps score well on the GIS scale. It all depends on what you put in them. Beans are a great low-GIS choice and are filling, so you'll have less room for dessert.
- Stick with the grilled seafood and chicken dishes such as fajitas or bean burritos, served with lots of crunchy salad and a fruity tomato or mango salsa. Avoid the sour cream and go easy on the cheese and guacamole. They may have a low GI but they are high in fat, so they aren't GIS-friendly.
- Watch out for the deep-fried taco salad shells — the word "salad" *doesn't* make it healthy, the word "fried" *does* mean high fat!
- Avoid the potato wedges: they're laden with calories, particularly when covered in melted cheese and sour cream. Ask for vegetable crudités or a plate of plain corn chips (5 GISs to share) with a spicy salsa tomato dip.

Remember Simple GI Diet Rule 2: *Stay as close as you can to your daily GISs.*

Breakfast at the "greasy spoon"!
Not the easiest place to find healthier low-GI choices, but here we show you how.
- Try poached eggs on unbuttered toast.
- Some cafés serve oatmeal or muesli with 2% milk for breakfast. These are great low-GI cereals to keep your energy levels up throughout the morning.

The party pooper

We've all been there—you get to a party and are faced with a table full of yummy buffet goodies. It's too tempting to resist and so easy to overindulge! But beware, those tiny nibbles—sausage rolls and mini-quiches—are usually loaded with calories, and you're less conscious of the calories piling up since they look so small. What do you do?

- Have a low-GIS snack before you get there.
- Reach for the seeded bread or mini pita sandwiches. Choose those that aren't dripping in mayo. Roast chicken and salad, tuna and corn or ham and mustard are fine.
- Chicken drumsticks without the skin score well.
- If you're lucky, there will be a plate of crunchy salad vegetables and a dip. Have plenty of these but make sure you can still see the carrot when it comes out of the dip! Go for salsa and yogurt dips.
- Having made your choices, start circulating. You'll be so busy yapping you won't have time to eat!

Sensible drinking

Alcohol is very high in calories. An average glass of wine contains more calories than a banana. A shot of hard liquor has more calories than a packet of mints. A pint of beer has more calories than a small bag of potato chips. So, when eating out, watch the amount you drink, since the calories soon rack up.

- Drink GIS-free water or a diet soft drink before drinking any alcohol, so that you are not thirsty when you start.
- Ask for a pitcher of water with your meal and drink water between each sip of your alcoholic drink.
- Dilute alcohol, for example by mixing white wine with soda water to make a spritzer.
- Make sure you have diet drink mixers.

You may feel that choosing a healthy lifestyle means your days of having a quick drink with friends or a glass of wine over dinner are numbered. Our general philosophy is nothing is out of bounds. The key is balance, and making the right choices for you. Today's choices become tomorrow's consequences. And should you indulge in two or three drinks too many, you can count on your body letting you know, in no uncertain terms!

There's no reason why you cannot enjoy a drink (unless of course you have been advised to avoid alcohol for medical reasons), as long as you make sensible choices and drink in moderation. On the Simple GI Diet, the ideal amount is no more than seven units per

1 unit of alcohol = 1/2 pint (about two-thirds of a bottle) of beer = 1 standard glass of wine = 1 shot (about 1 ounce) of hard liquor, sherry, aperitif or liqueur.

week for a woman, and 10 units for a man. Alcohol does add calories, some drinks more than others, so the less you drink, the better for your target weight. Follow these guidelines:

- Avoid drinking on an empty stomach.
- If you enjoy hard liquor, mix single shots with sugar-free or low-calorie mixers.
- Avoid alcopops and creamy cocktails.
- Choose red wine. Studies have shown that the phenols in red wine increase levels of good cholesterol, and may help prevent blood clots and protect against heart disease.

Alcohol: maximum of 7 units for women, 10 units for men per week, in addition to your daily GISs.

On the move with fast food

Fast-food restaurants and cafés can spell trouble, but it doesn't mean they're out of bounds.

When a burger calls ...

- A hamburger bun has a higher GI value than seeded bread, so you get 5 GISs in the bun alone. Add one standard burger and it adds up to 8.5 GISs. Words like jumbo, giant, deluxe or supersized mean larger portions, larger GISs and larger hips. Order a regular hamburger (no cheese) or a kids size instead.

- Always say "no" to cheese.
- Veggie doesn't necessarily mean virtuous. Veggie burgers are generally still cooked in fat and served with a creamy sauce.
- Fries rack up 6 on the GIS scale. Thin-cut fries absorb more fat than thick ones, since there is a larger surface area for the oil to seep into. A "regular" portion instead of "large" could save you half the calories. Ideally, avoid fries if you can.
- Try adding a green salad—avoid the dressing and it's GIS-free. Remember v,v,p,c.
- Do your belly a favor and choose diet drinks—you can save yourself around 10 teaspoons of sugar by ordering a diet drink instead of a regular one.
- Munch through an apple or banana *before* you stop by, or order fruit chunks or fresh fruit, if available.

Sandwiches

At your local café or convenience store, sandwiches are readily available and are a quick and easy lunchtime option.

- Opt for bread with seeds or grains.
- Choose lower-GI breads such as wholegrain breads, sourdough or rye bread.

When you become crystal clear about adopting and adapting to a healthy lifestyle, you increase the likelihood of succeeding.

- Choose low-fat fillings such as lean meat, chicken or fish with piles of crunchy salad.
- Say "no" to mayo. Flavor with freshly ground black pepper, mustard, pickles, chutney, salsa or lemon juice.
- Finish off with some fruit and a low-fat yogurt, two great low-GI desserts.

Spuds

Baked potatoes have a high GI but you can lower the GI of the overall meal by choosing lower-GI fillings:

- Ask for no butter.
- Good fillings include baked beans (with a small sprinkling of grated cheese if you need it); chili con carne with kidney beans; tuna and corn (no mayo); coleslaw and beans; cottage cheese and salad. See the Lunch Combos for GIS values of some baked potato meals (pages 87-88).

Once in a while you will have to choose foods that are not so healthy. When this happens, remember that one unhealthy meal is not a disaster. You are not going to pile on the pounds by eating this one meal. You can always compensate by making sure your other meals that day, or the day after, contain healthier low-GIS foods. Remember, eating out is all part of the fun Simple GI Diet lifestyle.

The GIS IQ Test

Question:

Are you conscious of the types of fat you eat?

Choice 1: I eat fatty meats and full-fat dairy products because I can't resist them.

It's fine to choose these foods, just watch how often you eat them. If you overdo such high animal-fat foods, you are more likely to gain weight and risk raised cholesterol.

Choice 2: I choose foods and cooking methods that are low in fat.

As part of an overall healthy lifestyle, these foods help you keep in shape and support your Simple GI Diet and general health.

Choice 3: I eat oily fish once a week.

The special omega-3 fats in oily fish protect against heart disease and are in keeping with your GISs. Consequently, choosing oily fish on a weekly basis simply reduces your risks of heart problems.

Results:

Choice 1: Eating as you've always done can only lead to the same results. If you don't like what you're experiencing, change it NOW!

Choice 2: Making well-informed choices today will shape your life tomorrow. Life is a building process—each small action has a cumulative effect.

Choice 3: Celebrate your choice here and keep reminding yourself of the rewards that this brings!

Summary
- Eating out is one of the continued pleasures of life on the Simple GI Diet.
- Your choices today will shape your life tomorrow.
- Choose lower-GI breads with low-fat fillings.

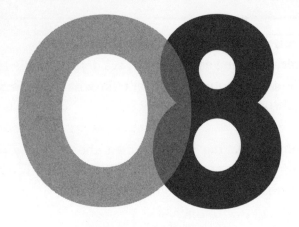

TASTY GIS RECIPES

Starters or side dishes

Baked Tiger Prawns
(1 GIS per serving)

You can use any type of shrimp or seafood for this dish, but tiger prawns add that special touch.

Serves 4

1 tbsp olive oil

2 cloves garlic, peeled and sliced thinly

*8 oz large raw shrimp (such as tiger prawns), peeled,
deveined and heads removed*

Garnish:

freshly chopped parsley

½ lemon, cut into wedges

1 Preheat the oven to 400° F.

2 Put the olive oil and garlic in a large, shallow, oven-proof dish and heat in the oven for 2–3 minutes until very hot. You need to watch this carefully so that the garlic does not start to brown.

3 Add the prawns carefully, rolling them in the hot oil, and return to the oven for another 3 minutes until they are pink and cooked.

4 Serve, sprinkled with freshly chopped parsley and lemon wedges.

Chili and Honey Chicken Wings
(2 GISs per serving)

Although this is basted with olive oil, the chicken wings are skinless, which helps to cut down on satu-rated fat. Finger-lickin' good, just remember to serve this dish with plenty of napkins!

Serves 4

12 skinless chicken wings
1 inch ginger root, crushed
2 cloves garlic, crushed
1 tsp red chili powder
1 tbsp olive oil
2 tsp honey
2 tsp coarse-grain mustard
1 tsp cider vinegar
salt and pepper

1 Preheat the broiler to medium. Line a large flame-proof dish with foil.

2 Put the wings into a bowl. Add all the other ingredients and mix well.

3 Arrange the chicken wings in the dish, making sure they don't overlap.

4 Cook under the broiler for about 20 minutes, turning once or twice during cooking. Serve hot or cold.

Beef Tomatoes with Black Olives
(1 GIS per serving)

Serves 4

8 beef tomatoes, sliced
12 pitted black olives, halved
paprika and garlic salt, to taste
1 tbsp olive oil
2 spring onions, sliced

1 Preheat the oven to 400° F. Lightly grease an oven-proof dish.

2 Layer the tomatoes with the olives in the dish and season with the paprika and garlic salt.

3 Drizzle on the olive oil and place on the middle shelf of the oven. Cook until soft but not mushy. Garnish with the spring onions and serve warm.

Middle Eastern Tabouleh Salad
(3 GISs per serving)

A Lebanese herby salad that goes well with kebabs and tzatziki (Greek yogurt with cucumber, garlic and mint) or with simple grilled fish.

Serves 4

3½ oz bulgur wheat, pre-soaked in
hot water for 1 hour, drained
3½ oz flat-leaf parsley, chopped roughly
5 medium tomatoes, diced
1 oz mint leaves (chopped)
1 oz coriander leaves (chopped)
1 medium onion, finely chopped

Dressing:
pinch of salt
pinch of ground allspice
pinch of ground cinnamon
juice of 2 lemons
2 tbsp olive oil

1 First make the dressing. Put all the dressing ingredients in a screw-top jar, cover and shake vigorously.
2 Mix the soaked wheat with the parsley, tomatoes, mint, coriander and onion.
3 Dress, toss and serve.

Kidney Bean and Chick Pea Salad in Mustard Dressing
(2.5 GISs per serving)

An unusual accompaniment to meat or fish—no need to add extra carbs since there are already some in the beans.

Serves 4

2 green bell peppers
1 oz fresh chives, snipped
6 spring onions, roots removed and chopped finely
7 oz can red kidney beans, drained
14 oz can chickpeas, drained
1 red onion, chopped

Dressing:

1½ tbsp olive oil
juice of 1 small lemon
1 clove garlic, peeled and crushed
2 tsp wholegrain French mustard
½ tsp mixed dried herbs

1 Spear the peppers with a fork and hold over a gas flame (or under a hot grill) until the skins are blackened all over.

2 Remove the skins and the seeds, then dice and place in a large bowl.

3 Add the chives, spring onions, kidney beans, chickpeas and red onion, and mix well.

4 Make the dressing. Put all the dressing ingredients in a screw-top jar, cover and shake vigorously.
5 Pour the dressing over the salad and mix well.
6 Cover and chill for at least 15 minutes before serving.

Chili Peanut Popcorn
(2.5 GISs per serving)

A crunchy snack for those curled-up-on-the-sofa video nights. Remember that this counts as your once-a-day nut allowance, so be sure not to have peanut butter or any other nuts on the same day.

Serves 3

2 oz salted peanuts
½ tsp red chili powder
½ tsp corn oil
2 tbsp popcorn
lemon juice, to taste

1 Heat a heavy-based pan with a lid, add the peanuts and toss them over medium heat until lightly toasted.
2 Remove from heat and place the peanuts in a bowl. While still warm, sprinkle with the red chili powder and stir well.
3 Pour the oil into the pan and, when heated, add the popcorn and cover. Maintain on medium heat. The corn should start to pop and hit the lid.

4 Remove from heat once the popping stops and pour the popped corn into the bowl with the peanuts. Stir well, add more chili powder if desired and lemon juice to taste just before serving.

(Recipe courtesy of the American Peanut Council.)

Main meals

Cod Kebabs with Fresh Dill
(1.5 GISs per serving)

Serves 4
1 lb 7 oz cod filet
1 tbsp olive oil
2 cloves garlic, crushed
zest and juice of 1 lemon
2 tbsp freshly chopped dill
2 tbsp freshly chopped coriander leaves
salt and black pepper
2 limes, quartered
cherry tomatoes

1 Cut the fish into chunks and place in a bowl with the olive oil, garlic, lemon zest and juice, dill, coriander and seasoning. Stir well.
2 Pre-heat the broiler to medium and line a grill pan with foil.

3 Thread the fish pieces onto four skewers and secure the ends with the lime wedges.

4 Grill, turning occasionally, for about 5–8 minutes. Serve with halved cherry tomatoes.

Salmon Steaks in Garlicky Balsamic Vinegar
(3.5 GISs per serving)

You can prepare this dish in the same amount of time as it takes to set the table—literally 5 minutes! The salmon is smothered in a mixture of fresh garlic, soy sauce, coarse-grain mustard and balsamic vinegar, and grilled quickly. (Alternatively, try wrapping the fish in aluminum foil with a sprig of fresh dill and some chopped spring onions, and cook in a moderate oven.) Serve on a bed of brown rice, with a crisp green salad, and for that really special occasion, partner it with asparagus tips.

Serves 4

4 salmon steaks, about 6 oz each
2 tbsp balsamic vinegar
2 tbsp soy sauce
1 tbsp olive oil
2 heaping tsp coarse-grain mustard
2 garlic cloves, crushed
2 tbsp fresh dill, finely chopped
salt and freshly milled black pepper

1 Place the salmon steaks in a non-metallic dish.

2 Mix together the vinegar, soy sauce, olive oil, mustard, garlic, dill and seasoning.

3 Pour the sauce over the salmon, turning to coat. If marinating, cover and leave in the refrigerator for 30 minutes.

4 Preheat the grill. Lift the salmon out of the marinade and place on a foil-lined grill pan. Coat the steaks with the sauce and grill over moderate heat for 4–5 minutes each side.

Haddock with Thai Green Pepper and Basil Sauce
(2.5 GISs per serving)

You can use any white fish for this dish, though haddock or cod fillets work especially well. The green pepper and basil are combined with a Thai green curry paste to make an unusual and exciting blend of flavors.

Serves 4

4 haddock fillets, about 6 oz each
1 tbsp olive oil
1 tsp crushed garlic
1 tsp crushed ginger
salt and coarse black pepper

Sauce:
3 green bell peppers, halved and de-seeded

2 tsp olive oil
1 onion, chopped
2 tsp Thai green curry paste
Few fresh basil leaves, torn
1 sprig of fresh thyme or a pinch of dried thyme
2 tbsp lime juice

Garnish:

Few sprigs of fresh coriander

1 Preheat the broiler. Place the peppers, skin side up, on a baking sheet. Cook under a hot broiler until the skins are blackened. Set aside to cool.

2 Now make the sauce. Heat the oil and sauté the chopped onions until translucent, about 2–3 minutes. Add the curry paste and cook for another minute.

3 Peel the peppers and place them in a food processor with the onion mixture, herbs and lime juice. Blend until smooth. Adjust the seasoning if necessary.

4 Brush the fish lightly on both sides with the olive oil, and sprinkle with garlic and ginger. Season and place on a foiled grill pan. Broil, turning once, until the fish flakes easily (about 10–12 minutes).

5 Serve the fish with the green pepper sauce, garnished with fresh coriander.

Turkey Stroganoff
(1.5 GISs per serving)

A low-fat version of the traditional stroganoff. Serve with basmati rice (remember to add the GISs) and a fresh herb salad.

Serves 4

Spray oil
1 lb 2 oz turkey breast, diced into chunks
2 small onions, thinly sliced
½ oz freshly chopped mint leaves
4 tbsp low-fat natural yogurt
salt and pepper
fresh coriander leaves, to garnish

1 Heat 5 sprays of oil in a non-stick pan and fry the turkey pieces until lightly colored.

2 Add the onions and stir the mixture until lightly browned.

3 Stir in the remaining ingredients and gently bring to a boil, stirring all the time to prevent curdling.

4 Cover and simmer on low heat until the meat is cooked. Season and garnish with coriander.

Beef Chow Mein
(7 GISs per serving)

This tangy dish is delicious for a special occasion or for an evening meal when you have those insatiable hunger pangs. The beef is cut into thin strips so it takes very little time to cook. Noodles and other pasta have a low Glycemic Index. Serve with lots of vegetables.

Serves 4

3 tbsp soy sauce
16 oz rump steak, cut into thin strips
1 inch piece ginger root, peeled and sliced
into thin strips
2 tbsp rapeseed oil
1 onion, thinly sliced
1 green or red bell pepper, cut into chunks
2½ oz button mushrooms
2 large tomatoes, cut into wedges

Noodles:
12 oz instant noodles
2 tsp rapeseed oil
salt and pepper

1 Drizzle the soy sauce over the beef, add the ginger and, if you have time, leave to marinate for 30 minutes. Drain the beef, reserving the marinade.
2 Cook the noodles in a large saucepan of boiling water, following the instructions on the packet. Drain and set aside.
3 Heat 2 tbsp rapeseed oil in a wok and stir-fry the meat for 2–3 minutes on high. Remove with a slotted spoon and keep warm.

4 Add the onion, pepper and mushrooms and stir-fry for 4 minutes. Next add the marinade, cooked beef and the tomato wedges. Cook for 2–3 minutes until the vegetables are cooked but crisp.

5 Heat 2 tsp of rapeseed oil in a wok or large pan. Stir in the noodles, season. Serve with the beef.

Couscous with Peppers and Red Onion
(4.5 GISs per serving, main meal; 2.5 GIS per serving, side dish)

Couscous makes a refreshing change from potatoes, rice and pasta. In this recipe, it is mixed with crunchy chopped peppers, flat-leaf parsley and red onion to give a flavorsome carb accompaniment to any meal.

It can be served hot or cold and can be bought in flavored varieties, such as lemon and garlic. This recipe can be made up to 24 hours in advance and kept covered in the fridge until needed.

Serves 4 as a main course, 6–8 as a side dish

8 oz couscous

4 tsp olive oil

juice of 1 lime

3 small mixed bell peppers, de-seeded and finely chopped

1 small red onion, finely chopped

1 bunch of flat-leaf parsley (about 3 oz), washed and roughly chopped (remove any tough stalks)

1 Put the dry couscous in a large mixing bowl.

2 Add the same amount of boiling water (8 fl oz) and stir briefly with a fork.

3 Stir in the olive oil and lime juice.

4 Add the chopped peppers, onion and flat-leaf parsley leaves and mix well.

5 Leave, out of the fridge, for 30 minutes for the flavors to develop and mingle.

Mediterranean Pasta
(5 GISs per serving)

The smell of fresh garlic...the crunch of lightly cooked vegetables ... the colors of the Mediterranean. This delicious Italian meal is a filling family favorite, which goes well with a simple green salad.

Serves 4

3 tbsp olive oil
1 green, 1 red bell pepper, diced
3 zucchini, sliced thinly, diagonally
1½ tsp dried oregano
2 bay leaves
3 medium tomatoes, cut into eighths
8½ oz dried pasta (penne, for example)
3 cloves garlic, crushed
1 onion, finely chopped
1 lb mushrooms, sliced

salt and coarsely ground black pepper
1 tbsp fresh parsley, finely chopped

1 Preheat the oven to 475° F. Drizzle a teaspoon of oil into a large roasting pan. Layer the peppers and zucchini into the pan, adding the oregano, bay leaves and seasoning in between the layers. Drizzle the remaining oil over the vegetables, saving about two teaspoons of oil for the pasta.

2 Bake uncovered at the top of the oven for 20–25 minutes, until slightly charred, adding the tomatoes after about 15 minutes. Stir once during cooking.

3 Cook the pasta in lightly salted water according to the instructions on the package.

4 Meanwhile, heat the remaining oil in a large non-stick pan. Add the garlic, onion and mushrooms and fry until the onions are light brown and the mushrooms are just cooked.

5 Take the vegetables out of the oven, stir gently. Mix thoroughly with the pasta and mushroom-and-onion mixture. Adjust the seasoning if necessary, and sprinkle with parsley.

Speedy GIS-free snacks

Garlic Mushrooms

Put some button mushrooms into a pan with low-sodium soy sauce, garlic purée, cracked black pepper and any dried herbs you have lying around. Throw in chopped spring onions or chives. Cook quickly and eat slowly.

Cabbage with Fennel Seeds

Steam some cabbage, or raid the fridge for leftover GIS-free vegetables. Warm a frying pan and pour in a little balsamic vinegar. Add the cabbage, a teaspoon of fennel seeds, a pinch of cayenne pepper, a touch of salt and some ground black pepper. Cook until tender.

Grilled Tomato Salad

Slice a large tomato, season with paprika and garlic salt. Place under a preheated grill until charred. Remove, and top with chopped red onion.

Zucchini Boats

Cut a zucchini in half lengthwise. Flavor with black pepper, ground cumin or curry powder. Add a little salt and some lemon juice. Microwave on high until just cooked—about a minute or so.

Chili and Lime Arugula Leaves

Mix together your favorite combination of GIS-free salad veggies and arugula leaves. Make a dressing using fresh lime juice, paprika, dried herbs and chili sauce. Drench and devour.

Yellow Squash and Leek Soup

Throw together about five ounces of chopped yellow squash, diced red peppers and leeks. Heat a pan with ½ pint of water and throw in half a stock cube (or less). Add the vegetables with a large pinch of dried parsley. Cook through, remove and add pepper to taste.

Savoy Cabbage with Caraway Seeds

Steam about 5 oz cabbage quickly until just cooked. Drain. Add five sprays of spray oil to a non-stick frying pan. Heat the oil and add the cabbage. Stir-fry over a high heat with a teaspoon of caraway seeds. Season, sprinkle on some cayenne pepper and serve.

Herby Baby Spinach and Beansprouts

Simply mix the spinach and beansprouts together and flavor with fresh flat-leaf parsley, rice vinegar and paprika.

Gherkin and Onion Pickle

Chop some gherkins; add a halved pickled onion or two, sprinkle with red chili powder.

Stir-fried Baby Corn

Heat a pan with five sprays of oil. Add baby corn. Season with a little soy sauce and black pepper. Cook until heated through.

Curried Okra

Heat five sprays of spray oil and add a good pinch of cumin seeds. Let them pop for a few seconds over a low heat to release the aroma. Add a couple of teaspoons of tomato purée and a good pinch of curry powder. Blend together over a low heat—add some water if it sticks to the bottom. Toss in around six pieces of boiled or canned okra and some diced red onion or spring onions. Cook until tender. Smother in freshly chopped coriander.

Balsamic French Beans

Boil French beans until just cooked. Drain. Add balsamic vinegar and a little salt to taste.

Roasted Vegetables

Mix together your favorite combination of chopped bell peppers, mushrooms, onions, zucchini, asparagus, celery, baby corn and tomatoes. Add a teaspoon or so of crushed garlic, some fresh or dried herbs, a little salt and pepper. Place in a foil-lined tray and bake in a hot oven until cooked (about 15 minutes).

Speedy Salsa Sauce

Heat five sprays of spray oil in a non-stick frying pan and add a crushed clove of garlic. Stir-fry some finely chopped onion and green or red bell pepper. Add a couple of chopped canned tomatoes with some of the tomato juice and flavor with a good pinch of red chili powder. Simmer for about 5 minutes.

Cucumber and Mint Cooler

Cut some chilled cucumber into wedges and top with chopped fresh mint, lemon juice and coarsely ground black pepper.

Spiced Vegetables

Choose your favorite GIS-free raw or cooked vegetables and add a good pinch each of curry powder, paprika and ground cumin with a touch of salt.

Al Dente Asparagus

Steam asparagus tips with a little crushed garlic until lightly cooked. Season lightly and serve immediately.

Wheat-free Tabouleh

First make the dressing. Put a pinch each of salt, ground allspice and ground cinnamon and some lemon juice into a screw-top jar, cover and shake vigorously. Then make the tabouleh. Mix together some roughly chopped flat-leaf parsley, a couple of diced tomatoes, chopped mint leaves and a finely chopped onion. Toss in the dressing and serve.

Jell-O with Whole Strawberries

Make up a sugar-free Jell-O and add a cupful of fresh strawberries before the Jell-O sets completely. Leave to set and chill in the fridge. Alternatively, buy an individual container of sugar-free Jell-O, cut it into rough chunks and serve with fresh strawberries.

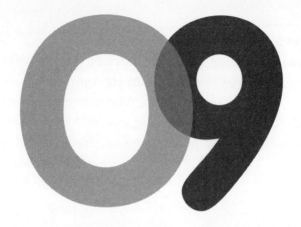

EATING FOR COMPLETE HEALTH

The balance of good health

The Simple GI Diet is your new way of life and, for it to be balanced and sustainable, it is crucial to include foods that provide the range of nutrients that enhance your overall sense of vitality and well-being. And since feeling great isn't only about what's on your plate, this chapter helps you incorporate other aspects of feeling good that are practical enough for the whole family.

Read on for a simple guide to which foods are good for you and why. You'll find lots of healthy eating tips, so just pick out the changes that you feel will easily fit into your lifestyle. Indeed, you may find that you are already choosing many of the recommended foods, so eating well may be easier than you think.

What are the five food groups?

- Bread, cereals (such as breakfast cereals) and starchy foods (such as potatoes, pasta and rice).
- Fruit and vegetables.
- Dairy products, such as milk and cheese.
- Meat, fish and alternatives, such as soy, beans and nuts.
- Fatty and sugar-laden foods.

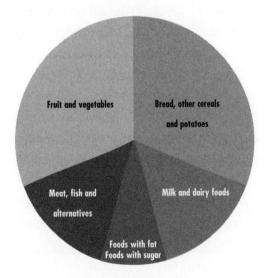

Remember Simple GI Diet Rule 8: *Choose a balanced diet by having a variety of foods from the different food groups.*

Bread and starchy foods

Love your carbs? No problem. You can devour them on this diet—from tortillas to fettuccine, since low-GIS carbs are all part of that buffet.

Starchy foods, such as bread, rice, potatoes and pasta, are great energy providers. GIS eating has the added benefit of pointing you to those starchy foods that are more likely to give you a slow, steady rise in blood glucose. These "right carbs" not only give you energy but also fill you up. That's because these foods take longer to digest, so you don't feel the need to reach for that extra helping or raid the fridge later.

Carbs also provide a wide range of vitamins, minerals and dietary fiber. Carbs can even be a good source of protein. You don't usually think of bread as a protein-rich food, but two slices of bread provide a significant proportion of your daily protein needs. And since protein foods help to stem your appetite, low-GIS protein foods, like beans, make even more sense.

At one time, carbs may have been thought of as the villains, since many people assumed these foods were fattening. In fact it's not the starchy foods that make

There's no need to think that there are foods you must eat and those you must not. Healthy eating is all about balance—choosing a variety of healthy foods you enjoy and not forcing yourself to eat foods you dislike.

you put on weight but the fatty toppings, dressings and sauces you serve with them. So, grainy bread is a great choice, but smother it in butter and it ends up on your hips or belly.

Some recipes in this book contain pasta, which is an excellent starchy food for Simple GI Dieters. Pasta is slowly absorbed by the body, so that it will not raise your blood glucose levels too quickly. If you keep an eye on added fat while cooking, this will mean even more success on your bathroom scales. When you've exhausted the range of things you can do with pasta and noodles there's still basmati rice, couscous, bulgur wheat, oats, sweet potatoes, yams, chapatis, tortillas and much more to sink your teeth into.

You can have virtually any carbs you like as long as you pay attention to the GISs. For example, if you're a potato addict, you'd do well to choose boiled new potatoes in their skins (3 GISs) rather than a baked potato (7 GISs). Similarly, basmati rice would come to the top of your shopping list when you're making a curry or Chinese meal. If you can find Bangladeshi rice (1.5 GISs) that's even better. Here are some more GIS tips:

Hints and tips

- Serve some low-GIS carbs at every meal. Remember that adding butter or margarine uses up more GISs.

- Fill your pantry with low-GIS choices such as tortilla wraps and seeded breads (like multigrain or sunflower seed bread).
- Experiment with a wider range of starchy vegetables such as yams, sweet potatoes and plantains.
- Try basmati rice and couscous for a change.
- Most types of pasta are low in GISs — make these your regular buddies. Keep the sauce simple. Tomatoes, onions, garlic and peppers don't need much more than a sprinkling of Parmesan cheese and freshly ground black pepper.
- Think "right carbs."

The fiber fill-up

Wholegrain varieties of bread and cereals as well as the skin on potatoes are high in fiber. High-fiber starchy foods, such as bran-based cereals and stone-ground whole wheat bread, also help prevent constipation. A simple way of checking if you're eating enough fiber is to check your stools! If they float in the toilet bowl you're okay; if not, try a bowl of wholegrain breakfast cereal a day and more fruit and vegetables, drink lots of water, and watch 'em float over the next few days.

It's important to drink plenty of water to help the fiber do its job. Try to have at least six to eight glasses of fluid (such as water or low-calorie drinks) each day.

Oat-based cereals such as oatmeal and muesli are high in a particular type of fiber called soluble fiber.

These foods are even more slowly absorbed than starchy foods in general, which means they are ideal in GIS-eating. What's more, research shows that they can help reduce blood cholesterol. Try to use oats in recipes or start the day with an oat-based cereal. Instant hot oat cereals do contain soluble fiber, but because the oats have been mashed up, they raise blood glucose more rapidly than other types. Go for oats with large flakes instead.

Remember Simple GI Diet Rule 1: *Eat three meals and three snacks every day.*

Spread your intake of starchy foods evenly throughout the day and eat regular meals and snacks. This helps to reduce fluctuations in your blood-glucose levels.

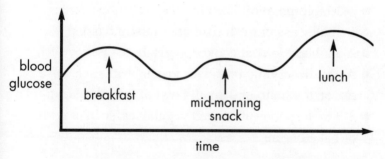

Fruit and vegetables

What do you do if your get-up-and-go just got up and went? Well, the answer is "Give me five" — fruit and vegetables, that is. In fact, this advice makes so much sense that you'll not only experience a boost of vitality, the extra vitamins and minerals you take in will help build a sound nutritional barrier against cancer and other diseases. And the best news is that most fruit and vegetables are low in GISs. Weight loss never tasted so good!

How much is enough?

For good health, you should aim for five three-ounce portions a day. (Potatoes are classified as starchy carbohydrates, so they don't count.)

What's in a portion?

- Medium apple, pear, orange or banana
- Large slice of melon or pineapple
- 5 oz of strawberries or grapes
- ½–1 tablespoon of dried fruit
- 1 small glass of fresh fruit juice (about 5 oz)
- 2–3 tablespoons of cooked vegetables
- A small serving of salad vegetables, such as a carrot, a tomato or a small bowl of mixed salad
- 2–3 tablespoons of canned vegetables, such as corn or baked beans

What about juice, dried fruit and veggies in pre-packaged meals?

As you can see from the list, dried fruit and fresh fruit juice do count. However, it is best to choose juice as only one of your five portions, since the valuable fiber

Dark green fruit and vegetables

Vitamin A	Cabbage, broccoli, spinach, lettuce, parsley and green peppers
Vitamin B	Cabbage, broccoli, spinach, green peppers, watercress and parsley
Vitamin E	Broccoli, spinach, green peppers, watercress and parsley
Vitamin K	Most green leafy vegetables
Calcium	Most green leafy vegetables
Iron	Spinach, watercress and parsley
Potassium	Broccoli, spinach, green leafy vegetables

Yellow and orange fruit and vegetables

Vitamin A	Carrots, tomatoes, red peppers, apricots, mangoes, cantaloupe
Vitamin C	Oranges, lemons, grapefruit, kiwi fruit, mangoes, strawberries, blackberries, black currants, cranberries, tomatoes, red and green peppers
Calcium	Black currants and blackberries

has been removed. And since juice generally makes your blood glucose rise more quickly than the whole fruit, it's best to have it with a meal so that the rise is evened out by other foods eaten at the same time. Legumes (such as beans and lentils) are also counted just once a day. This is because they don't contain the range of nutrients you get from other foods such as green leafy vegetables, carrots and tomatoes.

So, about half a can of baked beans counts as a portion, and interestingly, since there might well be three ounces of tomatoes in a portion of tomato-based pasta sauce or three ounces of vegetables in a packaged stir-fry, then you can, in theory, achieve your five-a-day target by eating packaged foods. However, it makes good nutritional sense to have a mixture, to be sure of getting all the nutrients you need, especially since processed foods are usually high in salt. Check out the Smart Shopping chapter (page 53) for some low-GIS fruit and veggies.

If you're not wild about cabbage and broccoli don't despair. It's all about variety and choosing foods you enjoy. For example, try using a thin pizza crust and smothering it in spinach, peppers, tomatoes, onions and garlic. Fruit smoothies made with 2% milk are another great way to get an extra couple of portions of fruit in.

"Antioxidants"—that magic word

These are natural substances found in fruit, vegetables and some nuts. They include vital vitamins such as vitamins A, C and E as well as lycopene (concentrated in tomatoes), flavenoids (found in tea) and the mineral selenium (found especially in Brazil nuts).

Antioxidants are thought to be protective since they "mop up" the free radicals, which lurk around in the body and have been linked to premature aging, heart disease and cancer. Free radicals are produced by normal body processes, but cigarette smoke, ultraviolet light, illness and pollution appear to increase their production. Vitamins have many other health-giving properties. For example, vitamin E can help to strengthen the blood vessels. Vitamin C helps you to absorb iron, which is needed for healthy red blood cells and to prevent anemia, so have a couple of mandarin oranges or other citrus fruit after a meal that contains iron-rich foods such as meat or broccoli.

And the antioxidant lycopene, concentrated in tomatoes, becomes more potent when the tomatoes are processed. So smothering pasta with a jar of tomato-based pasta sauce might be cheating in the kitchen, but be smug that your meal is packed with hidden benefits. And mixing a chunky sauce with low-GI boiled pasta helps you to keep the GI low.

Rainbow eating
The brightly colored red, yellow and orange veggies are particularly rich in antioxidants, especially beta-carotene. Packed with cancer-fighting power, these "phytochemicals" are present in fresh fruit and vegetables in precisely the quantities and combination Mother Nature intended. So taking a vitamin containing one or two of them just won't do the trick, compared with the combination found in real foods.

Get into the habit of surveying the natural colors on your plate—the more varied the colors, the more varied the nutrients. Easy as pie! Generally speaking, dark or colorful fruit and vegetables contain more goodness than paler ones, but they're all worth including so you get a good mix.

When is a legume not a vegetable? When it's a peanut!

Believe it or not, the peanut is actually a legume, and studies show that about one ounce a day can be protective against heart disease and cancer. Although they are very similar to beans and lentils, their nutritional make-up is very different. Throw in a handful to enhance a stir-fry or salad, or slap some peanut butter and banana on bread for a tasty sandwich. Since, like most other nuts, they are lower in GISs than you might expect, scattering a few on to your plate will help to lower the overall GI of the meal (unsalted nuts are best). Remember, though, that they are high in calories, so don't exceed one ounce (a small handful) a day.

Hints and tips

- Eat five servings of fruit and vegetables every day. Remember that fruit juice can count as one of these servings but the GI will be higher.
- Buy fresh fruit and vegetables often and choose the highest quality that fits your budget, and ideally

the firmest.

- Vegetables are generally low-GIS foods—aim to fill at least half your plate with them at main meals.

- Try to eat a salad or some fresh fruit at each meal. Skip salad dressings to keep the calories down, unless they're fat-free.

- Experiment with meals that are made up completely of raw food. You might enjoy the crunch and wholesomeness. Remember rainbow eating.

- Very often vitamins and minerals are concentrated just under the skin so scrub rather than peel potatoes, carrots and apples.

- Rather than leaving fruit or vegetables standing in water, where they lose more vitamin C, chop or slice them just before cooking.

- Go for frozen vegetables—they can often be fresher than fresh vegetables. Supermarket fresh vegetables are rarely picked the same day.

- Serve vegetables as soon as they're cooked.

Dairy products

This group includes milk, cheese and yogurt. Dairy foods are excellent sources of calcium, and they also provide protein and vitamins. Calcium is vital for strong bones and teeth. Your bones are constantly being renewed and replaced, and right now you're probably not sitting on the same bones you were

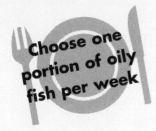

Choose one portion of oily fish per week

about seven years ago! Indeed children replace their skeleton roughly every two years. So you need a constant supply of bone-building nutrients to prevent your bones from becoming weak in later life. Physical activity is also essential for strong bones. See Chapter 10 for tips on being more active.

Full-fat dairy foods can be high in saturated fat. Too much of this type of fat may lead to raised blood-cholesterol levels, which in turn can increase your risk of heart problems. The GIS system takes this into account by offering you lower-saturated-fat versions of these foods. Aim for three different servings from this group each day to reach your recommended calcium levels. One serving is equivalent to about seven ounces of milk, five ounces of yogurt or a small matchbox-size piece of cheese. GISs have been allocated according to these serving sizes.

Vitamin D is needed to make use of the calcium in the foods you eat. Dairy products generally contain both vitamin D and calcium, so you get both nutrients at the same time. The body also makes vitamin D through the action of summer sunlight on the skin. Once made, vitamin D is stored in the liver for use during the winter.

Hints and tips

- Adults and children over five can choose skim or 2% milk in place of whole milk.
- Try low- or reduced-fat hard and soft cheeses. Check the labels to find those that are lowest. Medium-fat cheeses include Camembert, feta and mozzarella.
- Watch out for thick/creamy or Greek-style yogurts, which are higher in fat (but they are still better than cream).
- Choose a variety of dairy foods so that your three servings ideally come from different foods every day.

Meat, fish and alternatives

This group includes red meat, poultry, fish, eggs, legumes, soy products (such as tofu), nuts and seeds. These foods are rich in protein and many are good sources of vitamins such as A and D, and minerals such as iron and zinc. Protein provides the building blocks for growth and repair of the body. In addition, most of the important chemicals in the body, including hormones such as insulin, are made of protein.

There is some research to show that protein foods reduce appetite, so you'll find that moderate amounts of protein are recommended in the GIS plan. Choosing home-cooked foods (such as grilled chicken breast), rather than a prepared chicken meal (such as store-bought chicken casserole), will generally ensure that you get less salt and fewer additives. Too much protein can place a strain on the kidneys as they struggle to get rid of the waste products formed by the breakdown of protein. Choose two to three portions of protein foods a day, staying with the amounts as suggested in the GIS Table.

To reduce your saturated-fat intake, choose lean cuts of meat and minimize the fat you use in cooking. Processed meats such as burgers, hot dogs, sausages and smoked meats tend to be higher in salt and fat, so try to keep these foods to a minimum.

Opt for fish and vegetarian sources of protein as well as lean meats so that you get a variety. Vegetable proteins are also rich sources of fiber, vitamins such as folate, and antioxidants. You can make meat dishes healthier by adding beans or vegetables to recipes. This adds fiber, makes the meal go further and provides fewer calories per plate. What's more, since beans and vegetables tend to have a lower Glycemic Index, adding them to casseroles and stews helps to keep your blood glucose steady, giving you energy for longer.

Oily fish

There is good evidence to show that oily fish can protect the heart, even in people with established heart disease. One of the most notable studies was the British Diet and Reinfarction Trial, published in 1989, which studied 2,033 men under 70 years of age who had previously suffered a heart attack. One group increased their fish intake by eating two ounces of oily fish per day, which was three times higher than the other group. The results showed that

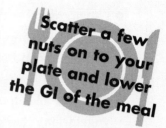

there was a 29 percent reduction in deaths, mostly those associated with coronary heart disease. In countries such as Japan, where people eat a lot of oily fish, the rates of heart disease are correspondingly low. Fish oil supplements have also been shown to have desirable effects on the heart.

The vital ingredient in oily fish is a fat called omega-3 and it is found in fish such as mackerel, herring, trout, tuna, salmon and sardines. Current advice is to choose one portion of oily fish per week. Some eggs are now enriched with omega-3 fats, so if you're not a fish lover, this might be a helpful source for you. You also get some omega-3 in soy beans and flaxseed.

Hints and tips

- Select lean cuts of meat and trim off visible fat.
- Cook meat without adding fat. For example, grill, roast on a rack, microwave, barbecue, poach, dry-fry and braise.
- Avoid using the juices from roast meat for gravy.
- Remove the skin from poultry.

- Use spray-oil and a non-stick pan for stir-frying.
- If you're opting for a vegetarian diet, remember that cheese and pastry can boost the fat content.
- Eat oily fish once a week.
- Nuts are an important source of protein if you are vegetarian. Recent research suggests that eating one ounce (about a handful) of nuts such as almonds around five times a week may help protect against heart disease.
- Add canned beans or chickpeas to soups and stews.
- Eat eggs poached, boiled or scrambled instead of fried. Limit to five or six eggs per week.
- If you rely on lots of convenience foods, look for low-fat and low-salt versions of pre-packaged meals.
- Marinade and stir-fry some tofu for a low-fat protein alternative.

Fatty and sugar-laden foods

This group includes spreads, dressings, oils, fries, chips, pastries, rich sauces, sugar, confectionery, sugary drinks, jams, cakes and cookies. Some fat provides essential fatty acids and vitamins. We even need some body fat for the protection and insulation of vital organs such as the heart and kidneys. However, we don't need all that much.

The whole issue of oils and fats can be confusing,

Alternatives to fat and sugar

Instead of ...	Try ...
Butter on bread	Grainy bread dipped in a little olive oil and balsamic vinegar
Corn oil in cooking	Rapeseed or olive oil
Sunflower oil in dressings	Fat-free dressings or a little walnut oil
Plain salad	Salad with a few added olives and walnuts
Sugar-coated breakfast cereal	Muesli, oatmeal, wholegrain cereals
Mayonnaise	Low-fat yogurt or fat-free dressings
Soft drinks	Unsweetened fruit juice, diet drinks or water
Rich frosted cake or doughnut	Plain crackers, oatmeal cookies
Rich desserts	Low-fat fruit yogurt, reduced-calorie ice cream, fresh fruit, canned fruit in natural juice, sugar-free Jell-O, reduced-fat pudding

for how can something be both bad and essential? We're told that high blood cholesterol is risky for the heart, yet foods high in cholesterol do not necessarily affect your blood cholesterol. Mediterranean eating gets the thumbs up, yet most of their salads swim in olive oil—how can this be?

In the Western world there is an abundance of fat-containing foods, and conditions such as obesity and heart disease are linked with a high-fat and high-calorie intake. So, boring though it may sound, moderation is always the key. Here are some home truths:

- Gram for gram, fat provides twice the calories of carbs or protein.
- Add fat and you bump up the calories. Fry an egg and the calories almost double, compared with a boiled or poached one.
- Fatty foods are often high in sugar too—think of Danish pastries and chocolate.
- Cooking oil has more fat and calories than butter, regardless of whether it's olive oil or corn oil.
- Some fats, such as omega-3, are essential, and you need a regular supply from the food you eat. This is why foods like oily fish are so good for you.
- Your liver produces cholesterol irrespective of the cholesterol in your diet. So cholesterol from eggs and shrimp, taken as part of a healthy diet, may have little effect on your blood cholesterol.
- You need fats to transport certain vitamins (fat-soluble ones) around the body.

Since we know that you will only lose weight if you take in fewer calories, it makes sense to limit the amount of fat that you eat. You'll notice that high-fat foods tend to have higher GISs—this will encourage you to make healthier choices more often. Also, there is some evidence to show that calorie-dense foods such as burgers and fries tend to be less filling, so you are likely to overeat. The Simple GI Diet plan limits these and guides you towards low-GI and moderate-protein foods, which help to satisfy your appetite for longer. People in Western countries generally eat far more fat than they need. You'll notice that food labels offer guidance on how much fat you should aim for in a day. This works out at around 70 grams of fat per day for a woman and 95 grams per day for a man.

In theory, you could achieve your daily GIS target by choosing unwisely, for example eating mainly fatty foods. However, you would be breaking the GIS rules and not following the plan correctly. Also, this is un-likely to fill you up so you may end up actually eating more. As a result, you miss out on vital nutrients, become less healthy and may not lose weight. Therefore, as the Simple GI Diet rules state, opt for a variety of low-GIS foods as often as you can since these will be inherently healthier. It is therefore a good idea to get into the habit of comparing food labels for their fat content, so you can make choices that fit into this target. For more on this, see Smart Shopping, Chapter 4.

So healthy eating isn't necessarily about low-fat – it's about the *right* fat. Research shows that a mono-unsaturated-fat-rich diet, as eaten in Mediterranean countries, may be preferable to a low-fat diet. Don't get too excited.... This doesn't mean filling up on pastries and hot dogs, because they do not contain the right types of fats for good health. Monounsaturates are found in foods like olive oil, rapeseed oil, almonds and other nuts, and avocados. Though high in fats, they help you stay healthy and you may even lose weight in the right context. If you are a science addict, turn to page 228 for some research on this.

Since people who are overweight are at an increased risk of getting heart disease, watching your fat intake is particularly important. Eat less saturated fat, such as whole milk and cheese, fatty meat, hot dogs, pies and pastries.

Replace some of the foods that contain a lot of saturated fat with those that are high in mono- or polyunsaturated fat. For example, use small amounts of rapeseed, olive, corn or sunflower oil in cooking, and a scraping of butter on bread, or choose a reduced-fat spread based on these oils. There is now a wide variety of low-fat foods available in supermarkets. Use reduced-fat versions of dairy products, such as 2% or skim milk, half-fat Cheddar cheese and low-fat yogurt. Note that reduced-fat doesn't mean no-fat—so don't go gorging on them just because the label says it's lower in fat.

The sweet stuff

Sugar, quite simply, can rot your teeth. If that's not a turn-off, then consider the fact that it can make you pile on the pounds. Since sweet foods tend to be high in fat as well (chocolate or cakes, for example), they are not a good choice for Simple GI Dieters. Even more importantly, sugar in liquid form encourages your blood sugar to rise, so when you do want a sweet treat, think about the best time — such as after a low-GIS meal. As for how much, ask yourself what would be the minimum to help you curb that craving while still keeping to your Simple GI Diet rules.

Fructose and lactose are types of sugar that are absorbed more slowly and so tend to prevent sugar rushes and energy highs and lows. You get fructose naturally from fruits, hence it is often called fruit sugar. You can now buy fructose in some supermarkets, and it is significantly lower in GI than ordinary granulated sugar. Lactose is the sugar that comes from milk and milk products.

Sugar comes in many other guises. For example glucose, dextrose, maple syrup, golden syrup, honey, brown sugar, invert sugar, hydrolyzed starch and fruit juice. As with any ingredient, the higher up on the ingredients list on a package an item appears, the more of it there is in the food.

If you would like to use a sugar substitute, artificial sweeteners such as saccharin, aspartame or ace-sulphame K are available in most supermarkets. They are much sweeter than sugar so much less can be used, but some people find the taste off-putting. They are carbohydrate-free, so they don't raise your blood glucose. Sucralose (marketed as Splenda) is a sugar substitute that has been made from sugar. The GI for it is not available, but it has 2 calories per teaspoon (compared to 20 calories for sugar).

Hints and tips

- Swap fatty sauces and dressings for healthier options — try mixtures of lemon juice, vinegar, mustard or yogurt and throw in a few herbs and spices.
- Use healthier cooking methods such as grilling, baking, microwaving, poaching or stewing, instead of frying foods.
- Buy the leanest cuts of meat you can afford.
- Keep healthier snacks in your cupboard — the Snack Attack chapter (page 98) will have you oozing with ideas.
- Shop for monounsaturates, such as rapeseed oil, olive oil, nuts and seeds. And here's a bonus tip — rapeseed oil is much cheaper than olive oil, and is available in most supermarkets. Look closely at the label for rapeseed, as it is sometimes sold as vegetable oil.
- Consider bread without butter — do you really need it if you're going to be dipping the bread into soup, for example?

Acting out of well-informed choices today will shape your life tomorrow.

- Replace cream with low-fat or non-fat yogurt.
- Eat fruit instead of sweets—the fructose in fruit is less damaging to your teeth and blood glucose levels, compared to the sucrose in sweets.
- If you take sugar in tea or coffee, cut back half a teaspoon per cup each week. Your taste buds have an amazing way of adapting, so you'll find you get used to less sugar. Keep going and you'll cut out sugar altogether—better for the waistline and the teeth.

Salt

Salt is the common name for sodium chloride and it is the sodium part that is considered to be harmful if used in excess. On a food label, you may not see salt on the ingredient list, but that doesn't mean the food is sodium-free. Sodium can be listed in different ways, for example, monosodium glutamate, soy sauce, bicarbonate of soda, and when a food is "smoked."

Good sense with salt is one of the key health messages, as eating too much salt has been associated with high blood pressure and strokes. If you eat too much salt it's likely that your body will hang on to excess water, which can lead to symptoms such as bloating and swollen ankles.

It is recommended that we eat no more than six grams of salt (just over a teaspoon) a day. About two-thirds of the salt we consume comes from processed foods, such as bread, canned soups, breakfast cereals, sausages and savory snacks. (Even sweet foods may contain salt.) So check the labels carefully. If most of the salt you eat comes from manufactured foods, and if you are addicted to pre-packaged meals and fast

Salt content of some common foods

Food	Average sodium (grams)	Salt (grams)
Bread and cakes		
White bread—1 medium slice	0.2	0.5
Whole wheat bread—1 medium slice	0.2	0.5
Jelly doughnut—1	negligible	0.1
Fruit scone—1	0.4	1.0
Cheeses		
Cheddar—small matchbox-size piece	0.2	0.5
Stilton—small matchbox-size piece	0.4	1.0
Cottage cheese—2 tablespoons	0.4	1.0
Processed cheese—2 slices	0.5	1.2
Meat, fish and eggs		
Bacon—2 lean slices	1.1	2.7
Sausages—2 large	0.8	1.9
Ham—1 lean slice	0.3	0.7
Roast chicken—2 thick slices	negligible	0.2
Egg—1	negligible	0.2
Breakfast cereals		
Cornflakes—medium bowl	0.3	0.7

Salt content of some common foods

Food	Average sodium (grams)	Salt (grams)
Snacks		
Potato chips—25 gram bag	0.2	0.5
Peanuts, salted—50 gram bag	0.2	0.5
Peanuts, dry roasted—50 gram bag	0.4	1.0
Banana—1	negligible	negligible
Vegetables		
Corn on the cob— average serving, unsalted	negligible	negligible
Corn—average serving, salted	0.3	0.7
Peas—average serving, salted	negligible	0.2
Pasta		
Spaghetti in tomato sauce— ½ standard can	1.0	2.4
Macaroni and cheese—5 tablespoons	0.7	1.7

foods, you might be going overboard on the salt front.

Most food labels give you the amount of sodium, but the daily guidelines are based on the amount of salt. So, to work out the amount of salt in a food, you simply multiply the sodium figure by 2.5 (2.4 to be precise!). And since this is often per 100 grams of the food, you then need to figure out how much salt you get in a portion if the label doesn't tell you. Easy? Hmmm … We've done some of the calculations for you (see the table above) so you can compare some common foods.

Hints and tips

- Processed, convenience foods are often loaded with salt. These include hot dogs, bacon, some canned fish and smoked foods such as smoked fish. Instead choose fresh fish, meat, fruit and vegetables. Only a small amount of salt is present naturally.

- Cut down on salty foods such as chips, crackers and salted nuts. Choose fresh fruit, unsalted nuts and dried fruit as alternative snacks.

- Think about the amount of salt you add in cooking and gradually use less.

- Avoid adding salt at the table.

- Experiment with new flavors such as exotic herbs, freshly ground spices, freshly ground black pepper and paprika. Also try lime juice, balsamic vinegar and chili sauce. If you find it hard to adjust to less salt, try a salt substitute, which enhances the flavor without adding as much sodium. Low-salt products (such as tuna in water, canned vegetables in water, unsalted bread and butter) are available in supermarkets and can be used instead of salt-rich foods.

The GIS IQ Test

Question:

When you're watching your weight, what do you do?

Choice 1: Mostly, I eat regularly and in small amounts and I aim for a slow, steady weight loss. I really only eat when I'm hungry.

A weight loss of one to two pounds per week is the best way to ensure that the weight stays off! Eating six times a day is ideal for the Simple GI Dieter.

Choice 2: I'm currently making gradual changes to my lifestyle — healthy foods and regular exercise.

A tailored approach is great — the sure way to becoming thinner is to choose a plan that fits in with your lifestyle. Team this plan] up with regular physical activity and you've got it made!

Choice 3: I often try crash diets and milk-shake diets since they promise quick results!

There is no healthy way to lose weight fast. Such diets encourage a dieting mentality. Yo-yo dieting is more harmful to your health than being slightly overweight.

Results:

Choice 1: You'll appreciate a state of consistent high energy and a sense of overall well-being that will help you to sustain a positive mental attitude. This is likely to support you in reaching/maintaining your ultimate weight.

Choice 2: You've done the trickiest part! You're making important changes today. The choices that you make now will shape your life.

Choice 3: Change your thinking so that achieving your goal becomes pleasurable and fun. Let it become an enticing way of enriching your life. This way, you're likely to succeed long term, as opposed to quick-fix methods that don't necessarily last!

Summary

- The more varied the colors on your plate, the more varied the nutrients.
- Oatmeal and muesli are ideal in GIS-eating, as are legumes: choose them regularly.
- Most fruit and veggies are low in GISs: include five portions, daily.

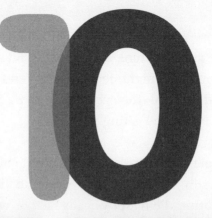

THE SIMPLE GI DIET LIFESTYLE PLAN

Get physical!

Is this you?

- Every day you look in the mirror and say, "If I lose a few pounds, I'll be happier, successful, more attractive …"

Simple GI Diet Rule 7:
Have at least two 10-minute bursts of moderate-intensity physical activity every day.

- You lose weight but you are still unhappy, because inside you still think of yourself as fat.
- You are overweight, feel unhappy and are finding it hard to break the cycle of yo-yo dieting and/or other unhealthy eating patterns.

The Simple GI Diet recommends short chunks of regular physical activity that are easy to fit into your daily routine. Being physically active while taking part in any weight-loss program is key to long-term success. If you can maintain some sort of regular activity (and this could be as simple as taking the dog for a brisk walk), it can help you keep the weight off once you reach your target. For exercise to be of lasting benefit, make it as regular as brushing your teeth and take it as seriously as your driving test.

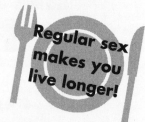

Regular sex makes you live longer!

Create the energy to exercise just by going for it. Too much thinking can slow you down! If much of your day is spent behind a desk, or in a stuffy environment, you may well feel lethargic and tired. In that case, moving around and getting some fresh air will have an even greater and more beneficial impact. Think about doing some physical activity as soon as you finish work or once you get home. Just 10 minutes can make a big difference.

Keeping fit is one of the best preventative medicines available to you, often at no extra cost. Whatever your age, a total of 30 minutes of moderate exercise five times a week is a great insurance policy. It can be as simple as a brisk walk divided into three 10-minute chunks. This equates to around 150 minutes of 10-minute slots each week. The Simple GI Diet recommends two 10-minute bursts a day, which is around 140 minutes per week. Try these:

- Walk farther to buy your lunch.
- Get off the bus or subway one stop before you need to and walk the rest of the way.
- Use the stairs when you can — ups are better than downs!
- Walk up *and* down escalators.
- Dance to your favorite music around the house: you can combine it with doing your daily chores. Even

Chart your activity progress

Use this chart to record how many of the 10-minute activity sessions you're doing each day. Simply pencil in a check mark every time, aiming for two checks per day.

	Mon	Tue	Wed	Thur	Fri	Sat	Sun
Week 1							
Week 2							
Week 3							
Week 4							
Week 5							
Week 6							

30 minutes of slow dancing knocks off the cals.

- Spend quality time with the children in a swimming pool or the park. This can be an energetic and fun way to engage with your kids.
- Walk the dog, or borrow a neighbor's! It's also a great way to make new friends.
- Play golf. It is an excellent way to drum up new business — work and play all rolled into one.

Feeling hot, hot, hot!

Here are some more quickies to get you started whether you're at home, in the office, car or bedroom. Yes, it is possible to burn off the calories and tone up without too much effort. The recipe to continued success is making exercise a part of your daily routine. Getting to a swimming pool can be hard work, as can going to the gym regularly. But there's lots of other things you can do. Get off those buns and get going! Here's how.

The home

- Gardening — you can burn off around 150 calories in half an hour of applying yourself to some spade work, for example.
- Running up and down stairs 10 times a day will eat

Find a form of exercise that you love and enjoy and build it into your daily routine.

up around 250 calories as well as helping you to tone the thighs and derrière.

- Ironing alone can use up to 150 calories in half an hour and vacuuming for around 30 minutes can help you lose another 200.

Household chores may no longer be a chore!

The office

- Park the car 10 minutes away or at the other end of the lot. A brisk walk to the office will help you burn off those calories.
- Instead of sending another dreaded e-mail, walk over to your colleague's desk.
- Ditch the elevator and take the stairs—two at a time when the need arises.
- Drinking plenty of water during the day is a must, so take regular walks to the water cooler or kitchen throughout the day. This will help you use up calories as well as keep you hydrated.
- Work on your feet! You'll burn calories by standing up and make your brain more alert. Do this hourly for several minutes at a time.

The car

- At the superstore, park as far away as you can from the entrance. Leave the shopping cart by the store so that you have to carry your bags back to the car, toning up along the way.

- If you're a parent, consider walking the kids to school instead of taking the car. You'll be less stressed and avoid the rush-hour congestion. Your children are likely to be more energized and alert when they start their day.
- Have you thought about buying a bike? One hour of cycling will help burn around 330 calories, and it will strengthen your lungs, heart, legs and back. Set aside the money that you save on gas and reward yourself in some way.

The bedroom

Just 30 minutes of sexy-cise will burn off around 200 calories. Sex is also said to lift your mood, reduce stress and boost your circulation. It's great for toning stomach and inner thighs. And if this fun, fitness and frivolity isn't enough, research tells us that regular sex makes you live longer.

All the activities suggested here will help you burn off those stubborn calories, but the amounts given can only be a general guide since everyone is unique.

Do try this at home!

Make a commitment to yourself. By looking after yourself, you ensure you will be there for others. Develop your lifestyle plan by going for simple bite-size chunks. This way, you're more likely to over-

Knowledge is not enough unless it is supported by a positive approach and mental attitude. By changing your thoughts you change your world, through choosing different actions.

achieve. You'll feel great, and your motivation will reach a momentum all of its own, since you know you can do it! Take a moment to think about what is truly important to you.

There are many, many reasons for making regular exercise a natural part of your daily routine. Here are some reminders about the benefits of exercise:

- Improves muscular strength and increases flexibility.
- Helps prevent varicose veins.
- Enhances your posture.
- Aids lower back pain and strengthens the spine.
- Helps to reduce anxiety, tension and stress.
- Enhances self-esteem and confidence.
- Helps prevent premature aging.
- Supports a balanced and healthy diet.
- Helps to beat the blues.
- Helps to keep up a healthy body image and good sex life.
- Burns calories.
- Reduces the risk of heart disease, osteoporosis and cancer.

And much more!

Switch your thinking

Even with the most effective dietary advice, your new way of eating might be short-lived unless you have prepared yourself mentally with a resourceful and positive mental approach. For the Simple GI Diet—indeed any lifestyle change—to be really effective, there are some key things to think about.

Many diets offer you weight loss if you avoid this and that food, but the more you're told to avoid it, the more you want it! Think back to when this might have been true for you. It's no wonder that you inadvertently sabotage the very goal that you set out to achieve by devouring the very food you're "not supposed" to have. Think about it. If you are programming your brain into thinking that a diet means food deprivation, your mind is likely to rebel against any diet before it's begun! So part of the trick here is to make the weight-loss goal as enjoyable, pleasurable and as much fun as possible.

Link pleasure to dieting and you'll be surprised how much easier it is to reach your happy weight in a safe and sustainable way. In your mind, connect this change with your choice of low-GI foods and a change in lifestyle, so that eating healthily becomes a natural, everyday part of your life. So, how do you transform pain into pleasure? Try our booster tips.

Booster tips

- Make a list of the long-term benefits that your new lifestyle will give you. For example, a general feeling of being well, an increase in self-confidence, looking and feeling great about yourself, a lowering of blood cholesterol and an increase in energy levels.

- Indulge and challenge your creative side! Think about the healthy, tasty foods that do it for you. Yes, that's right, you can have your cake and eat it too. Remember to choose foods that support you in reaching your goal, by focusing on the new you. Use our menu tips to put your own tailor-made eating plans together. Share them with family and friends. What you think about influences your behavior, so thinking and choosing more foods from the low- and medium-GISs section will naturally help you to attain that result faster.

- Take a moment to consider what's really important. Ask yourself this question: "Is the choice that I am making right here and now taking me closer to achieving what's truly important to me?" Whether it's the bar of chocolate, or the apple, that extra glass of something, or that eclair, choose wisely, knowing that different choices carry different consequences. Today's choices determine what happens tomorrow.

Motivational power booster

Here's one of the best-kept secrets! Working with the following exercise could change your life. Try it daily, as many times as possible, if you're ready to make those sustainable and long-lasting changes. Be careful what you think about, since you are highly likely to get it!

Imagine yourself as the "new" you that you most want to be. Study the picture in as much detail as you can, as if it has already happened. See yourself spending time with people who are supportive, fun and motivational. Visualize yourself being able to fit into your favorite jeans, being able to run after your kids (and catch them!), and doing things that previously you wouldn't have had the confidence to do.

Hear the comments others are making to you, now that you've achieved your goal. Hear their congratulations and other encouraging words. Say and repeat positive things to yourself, congratulating yourself on your achievements so far. What you say to yourself is key.

Feel the "positivity" of your success and how these feelings and emotions make you feel so great about yourself. Feel that enhanced sense of energy and inner confidence growing. Remember what this is doing for you and the difference that it is making to others close to you, too. Perhaps you are now enjoying new and varied interests with your family and loved ones.

Remember Simple GI Diet Rule 6: *Imagine the new you every day – a photograph will help.*

More steps to success

- If you do overindulge—enjoy it! This is not crazy advice. It frees you from feelings of guilt and anger, which make many people abandon their diets. Afterwards, simply get back on track.

- Keep a food and mood diary (see page 50) to show what you ate, where, why, and how you felt at the time. You may find that you eat in response to stress or strong emotions.

- Become more active. Walk to work instead of driving, use the stairs instead of the elevator, and take the dog for a walk.

- Try to make each meal an occasion to be enjoyed, sitting at the table, rather than stuffing down snacks at work or as you do the housework. Get into the habit of putting your fork down after every mouthful—it works wonders in helping you eat more slowly.

- Try to get your family and friends to support you. Tell them that you want to be thinner and healthier.

- Brush your teeth after every meal or snack—it really helps you stop eating.

- Write down your goal. Make it specific. For example, "I will weigh X on such and such a date."

- Believe in yourself. Know that you can *only* succeed. Keep a daily reference diary to record every success, no matter how small or large.

APPENDIX

THE GIS TABLES

Here is your list of everyday foods along with their GIS value. Entries are arranged in ascending order of GISs, and are split into the following groups:

- Meal carbs—choose one at each meal.
- Protein—choose two to three portions each day.
- Vegetables.
- Fruit.
- Drinks.
- Crackers and snacks.
- Seasonings.
- Fatty and sugar-laden foods.

On page 210, you'll find an alphabetical listing for quick reference—handy when you want to look up a particular food and you're in a rush.

The guidelines

1 The Simple GI Diet works because it helps to keep you full while you lose weight, and because it is based on a balanced range of healthy foods. In order to use the tables as they are intended, follow these simple guidelines:

- Eat three meals and three snacks every day.
- Choose fruit or other low-GIS foods for snacks.
- Stick with the instructions at the top of each section.

● Picture your plate in quarters and fill two quarters with vegetables (v, v), one quarter with protein (p) and one quarter with carbs (c)—remember: "veggie, veggie, protein, carbs."

2 Use the serving sizes to guide you—these are designed to fill you up and help you keep a watchful eye on nutrition. If you're cooking for more than one person, use what you need to cook, but make sure that what *you* eat is the portion size suggested.

3 Use GIS-free snacks *in addition* to low-GIS carbs, not instead of them.

4 We know that adding a low-GI food to a high one offers a reduction in the overall GI, which means your blood glucose levels will be more stable, and you are less likely to feel hungry. Remember to try our healthy protein and carb meal combos, which have been calculated to take this extra benefit into account (see Chapter 5.) And if you choose one of these combos, you enjoy a bonus reduction in GISs! If you were to simply add up the GISs of the individual foods, you would notice that the GISs are lower with the combos. That's because we've used a simple formula to take into account the benefit of combining foods: "high + low = medium." Always remember the golden rule of combining high-GIS carbs with low-GIS carbs.

5 Look for low-fat or reduced-sugar versions of the listed foods, since this will help you cut calories.

6 For good long-term health, keep fatty and sugary foods to a minimum.

7 If you are a whiz in the kitchen (or even if you're not), the GIS-free seasonings will give you a host of tempting ways to spice up plain foods—simply adding some chili sauce to chickpeas, or garlic to mushrooms—makes a tempting treat in seconds. If you find other flavorings that are virtually fat- and carb-free (check the label), go right ahead and add them to your list.

8 Remember the five-a-day fruit and veggie mantra. The GIS-free vegetables and easy snack concoctions will help you achieve this effortlessly.

9 You will always have a daily allowance of seven ounces of 2% milk over and above your daily GIS total, so you can use this in drinks and in cooking without adding any extra GISs.

Food	Portion Size	GISs	Special Comments

MEAL CARBS

(choose one at each meal)

BEANS AND LENTILS (all beans and lentils count once a day as one of your five fruit and vegetables. These are also protein foods and if you choose them as your protein, then choose another carb)

Food	Portion Size	GISs	Special Comments
Chili beans, canned	7 oz	1	
Navy beans, dried, cooked	5 oz	1	
Lentils, red, split, dried, cooked	5 oz	1	
Black-eyed peas, dried, cooked	5 oz	1.5	GI of some canned beans is not available
Butter beans, dried, cooked	5 oz	1.5	
Chickpeas, whole, dried, cooked	5 oz	1.5	
Pigeon peas, whole, dried, cooked	5 oz	1.5	
Pinto beans, dried, cooked	5 oz	1.5	
Red kidney beans, dried, cooked	5 oz	1.5	you can use a combination of beans in smaller portions for the same GISs.
Soy beans, dried, cooked	5 oz	1.5	
Baked beans, canned in tomato sauce	5 oz	2	
Mung beans, whole, dried, cooked	5 oz	2	
Red kidney beans, canned	7 oz	2	
Chick peas, canned	7 oz	2	great spiced up as a snack – add chili sauce
Chickpeas, split, dried, cooked	5 oz	2.5	
Fava beans, dried, cooked	5 oz	3.5	
Fava beans, canned	7 oz	4	
Fava beans, frozen, cooked	5 oz	4	

BREADS

Food	Portion Size	GISs	Special Comments
Barley bread	2 slices	3	
Corn tortillas	2 tortillas	3	
Wheat tortillas	1 wrap	3	
Multigrain bread	2 slices	3.5	whole grains are richer in B vitamins than refined grains

Food	Portion Size	GISs	Special Comments
Pumpernickel bread	2 slices	3.5	
Barley and sunflower bread	2 slices	4.5	
Rye bread	2 slices	4.5	
White bread, with added fiber	2 slices	4.5	
Hamburger buns	1 bun	5	
Pita bread	1 pita	5	wholewheat ones are higher in fiber
Chapatis, made with fat	2 small chapatis	5.5	
White bread	2 slices	5.5	
Wholewheat bread	2 slices	5.5	opt for stoneground since it is more coarse and thus has a lower GI
Bagels, plain	1 bagel	6	a low-GIS carb helps to reduce the GI of the meal
Melba toast, plain	2 toasts	7	
Taco shells, baked	1 shell	7	
Baguette	1 individual	9	a great food but a very high GI. Always eat with a low-GIS carb (like salad)

BREAKFAST CEREALS (see low-combo breakfasts, page 84)

Food	Portion Size	GISs	Special Comments
All Bran and 2% milk	5 tablespoons+ 7 oz	2	try it with sliced banana
Oatmeal, made with water	8 tablespoons of oatmeal	3	
Oatmeal, made with milk and water	6 tablespoons of oatmeal using 3 oz milk and water as required	3.5	you could try skim milk, 7 oz, instead. Use a little sweetener, honey or fructose if you like, add the GISs
Muesli, reduced sugar and 2% milk	3 tablespoons+ 7 oz	4	
Special K and 2% milk	5 tablespoons+ 7 oz	4	
Bran Flakes and 2% milk	4 tablespoons+ 7 oz	4	

Food	Portion Size	GISs	Special Comments
Muesli and 2% milk	3 tablespoons+ 7 oz	4	
Muesli, Swiss style, and 2% milk	3 tablespoons+ 7 oz	4	
Puffed Wheat and 2% milk	5 tablespoons+ 7 oz	4	
Instant oatmeal made with 2% milk	follow pack instructions 7 oz	4.5	a package at work could be a convenient breakfast
Shredded Wheat and semi-skim milk	2 biscuits+ 7 oz	4.5	
Cornflakes and 2% milk	5 tablespoons+ 7 oz	4.5	
Nutrigrain and 2% milk	5 tablespoons+ 7 oz	4.5	
Grapenuts and 2% milk	5 tablespoons+ 7 oz	4.5	
Raisin Bran and 2% milk	4 tablespoons+ 7 oz	4.5	
Rice Krispies and 2% milk	7 tablespoons+ 7 oz	5.5	

PASTA *(most pasta is very low in GI. Use 2 oz raw per portion. Remember to add GISs from sauces)*

Food	Portion Size	GISs	Special Comments
Fettucine, egg, cooked	5 tablespoons	1.5	
Spaghetti, white, cooked	5 tablespoons	1.5	
Spaghetti, whole wheat, cooked	5 tablespoons	1.5	
Macaroni, cooked	5 tablespoons	2	
Noodles, instant, cooked	5 tablespoons	2	
Linguini, thick, cooked	5 tablespoons	2.5	
Linguini, thin, cooked	5 tablespoons	2.5	
Noodles, rice, cooked	5 tablespoons	3	

RICE AND GRAINS *(keep rice grains whole rather than soft and mushy)*

Food	Portion Size	GISs	Special Comments
Rice, white, Bangladeshi, boiled	6 tablespoons	1.5	available from Asian grocers
Barley, pearl, cooked	5 oz	1.5	throw some into soups and stews

Food	Portion Size	GISs	Special Comments
Bulgur, cooked	5 oz	2	
Rice, brown, boiled	6 tablespoons	2.5	
Rice, white, basmati, boiled	6 tablespoons	2.5	
Rice, white, precooked, microwaved	6 tablespoons	2.5	
Rice, white, easy cook, boiled	6 tablespoons	3	
Rice, white, instant, boiled	6 tablespoons	3.5	
Rice, white, polished, boiled	6 tablespoons	3.5	
Rice, white, risotto, boiled	6 tablespoons	3.5	
Couscous, cooked	5 oz	3.5	a nice change from rice
Semolina, cooked dry	5 oz	4.5	
Rice, white, glutinous (sticky), boiled	6 tablespoons	7	
Rice, white, jasmine, boiled	6 tablespoons	7.5	

SOUPS

Food	Portion Size	GISs	Special Comments
Minestrone soup, dried	1 soup bowl	0	GI of only these packaged soups is available, but you can try other flavors
Tomato soup, dried	1 soup bowl	0.5	
Tomato soup, cream of, canned	1 soup bowl	1	
Instant noodle soup	1 soup bowl	2	
Lentil soup, dried or canned	1 soup bowl	2	

VEGETABLES—STARCHY (these are part of carbs since they are high in starch. Other vegetables are not—you can find these under "Vegetables")

Food	Portion Size	GISs	Special Comments
Plantain, boiled	1 plantain	1.5	
Yam, baked	size of a medium potato	1.5	
Yam, boiled	size of a medium potato	1.5	
Yam, steamed	size of a medium potato	1.5	
New potatoes, boiled	4 new potatoes	3	keep skins on
New potatoes, canned, drained	4 new potatoes	3	
Potatoes, boiled	3 egg-size	3	

Food	Portion Size	GISs	Special Comments
	potatoes		
Sweet potato, boiled	1 small potato	3	source of beta-carotene
Sweet potato, steamed or microwaved	1 small potato	3	
Sweet potato, baked	1 small potato	3.5	
French fries, straight cut, frozen, oven baked	6 tablespoons	5	choose 5% fat varieties
French fries, fast food outlet	6 tablespoons	6	
Instant mashed potato made with water	2 scoops	7	
Potatoes, baked	1 medium potato	7	
Parsnip, boiled	2 tablespoons	7	serve with low GIS veggies
Parsnip, roast	2 tablespoons	7.5	

Food	Portion Size	GISs	Special Comments

PROTEIN

(choose 2–3 portions a day)

BEANS AND LENTILS (all beans and lentils count once a day as one of your five fruit and vegetables)

Food	Portion Size	GISs	Special Comments
Chili beans, canned	7 oz	1	
Navy beans, dried, cooked	5 oz	1	
Lentils, red, split, dried, cooked	5 oz	1	
Black-eyed peas, dried, cooked	5 oz	1.5	
Butter beans, dried, cooked	5 oz	1.5	
Chickpeas, whole, dried, cooked	5 oz	1.5	
Pigeon peas, whole, dried, cooked	5 oz	1.5	
Pinto beans, dried, cooked	5 oz	1.5	
Red kidney beans, dried, cooked	5 oz	1.5	you can use a combination of beans in smaller portions for the same GISs
Soy beans, dried, cooked	5 oz	1.5	
Baked beans, canned in tomato sauce	5 oz	2	
Mung beans, whole, dried, cooked	5 oz	2	
Red kidney beans, canned	7 oz	2	
Chickpeas, canned	7 oz	2	great spiced up as a snack – add chili sauce
Chickpeas, split, dried, cooked	5 oz	2.5	
Fava beans, dried, cooked	5 oz	3.5	
Fava beans, canned	7 oz	4	great with red onion
Fava beans, frozen, cooked	5 oz	4	

EGGS (max 5–6 per week, try omega-3 types)

Food	Portion Size	GISs	Special Comments
Eggs, boiled	2 eggs	1.5	
Eggs, poached	2 eggs	1.5	
Eggs, fried	2 eggs	3	
Eggs, scrambled, with milk and 1 tsp oil	2 eggs	3	
Omelette, plain, made with 1 tsp oil	2 eggs	3	

Food	Portion Size	GISs	Special Comments
FISH *(choose fish twice a week, one being oily fish which is rich in omega-3 fats)*			
Cod, baked	1 filet	1	
Cod, grilled	1 filet	1	
Haddock, steamed or grilled	1 filet	1	
Lemon sole, steamed or grilled	1 filet	1	
Oysters	1 dozen oysters	1	shellfish are a good source of zinc, great for immune function
Flounder, steamed or grilled	1 filet	1	
Shrimp, canned in brine, drained	1 small pot	1	
Tuna, canned in brine, drained	small can	1	half the calories of canned in oil
Crab	2 tablespoons crab meat	1.5	
Haddock, smoked	1 filet	1.5	smoked foods are higher in salt, so limit amounts
Halibut, steamed or grilled	1 filet	1.5	
Lobster	2 tablespoons	1.5	flavor with lemon juice
Mussels	6 mussels	1.5	
Salmon, smoked	3 slices	1.5	a source of healthy omega-3 fats
Scallops, steamed	3 tablespoons	1.5	
Shrimp	5 oz	1.5	
Trout, steamed or grilled	1 fish	1.5	a source of healthy omega-3 fats
Fish sticks, cod, grilled	4 sticks	2	
Herring, grilled	2 filets	2	a source of healthy omega-3 fats
Salmon, pink, canned in brine, drained	small can	2	a source of healthy omega-3 fats
Salmon, steamed or grilled	1 steak	2	a source of healthy omega-3 fats
Sardines, canned in brine, drained	4 sardines	2	a source of healthy omega-3 fats
Mackerel, canned in brine, drained	small can	2.5	a source of healthy omega-3 fats

Food	Portion Size	GISs	Special Comments

MEATS

Food	Portion Size	GISs	Special Comments
Beef stew, made with lean beef	6 tablespoons	1.5	limit or avoid fat in cooking
Ham	2 slices	1.5	
Lamb, loin chops, grilled, lean	2 chops	1.5	
Rabbit, stewed	6 tablespoons	1.5	
Beef, sirloin joint, roasted lean	3 slices	2	
Beef, rump steak, lean, grilled	5 oz steak	2	cooked weight
Chicken, breast chunks or strips	6 tablespoons	2	
Chicken, roasted	3 slices	2	avoid the skin, breast pieces are lower in fat
Chicken, breast, skinless, roasted	1 medium	2	
Chicken, leg, skinless, roasted	1 medium	2	
Chicken, thigh, skinless, roasted	1 medium	2	
Chicken, wing, skinless, roasted	4 wings	2	see recipe, page 127
Chicken, drumstick, skinless, roasted	2 drumsticks	2	higher in fat than chicken breast
Duck, roasted	3 slices	2	avoid the skin
Kidney, lamb, sautéed	2 kidneys	2	
Liver, ox, stewed	3 tablespoons	2	rich in iron and vitamin B12
Pork, leg joint, roasted	3 slices	2	
Pork, loin chops, grilled, lean	1 chop	2	
Turkey, roasted	2 slices	2	you get three times as much if you use wafer-thin turkey
Beef, ground, stewed	6 tablespoons	2.5	choose lean beef
Beef, topside, roasted well-done, lean	3 slices	2.5	
Corned beef, canned	2 slices	2.5	watch the salt!
Liver sausage	1 slice	2.5	all sausages tend to be high in salt and very processed
Liver, lamb, sautéed	2 slices	2.5	rich in iron, great for the immune system
Oxtail, stewed	6 tablespoons	2.5	
Tongue, ox, stewed	2 slices	2.5	

Food	Portion Size	GISs	Special Comments
Veal, cutlet, sautéed	1 cutlet	2.5	use spray oil
Veal, filet, roast	1 filet	2.5	
Bacon, back, grilled	3 slices	3	GI of turkey bacon is not available, but they are a lower-fat choice
Beef sausages, grilled	2 sausages	3	GI of lower-fat sausages is not available, but they are a better choice
Lamb, breast, roasted, lean	3 slices	3	
Pork sausages, grilled	2 sausages	3	
Bacon, middle, grilled	3 slices	3.5	
Hamburgers, chilled/frozen, grilled	2 hamburgers	3.5	
Chicken nuggets	6 nuggets	4	

DAIRY AND SOY

Food	Portion Size	GISs	Special Comments
Soy milk, unsweetened	7 oz	0.5	soy protein is rich in phyto-chemicals, shown to reduce blood cholesterol
2% milk	7 oz	0.5	
Skim milk	7 oz	0.5	
Cottage cheese, plain, reduced-fat	5 oz	1	
Drinkable yogurt	7 oz	1	choose reduced calorie if available
Yogurt, low-fat, natural	5 oz	1	
Cheese, ricotta	5 oz	1.5	
Cottage cheese, plain	5 oz	1.5	
Soy yogurt, fruit	5 oz	2	
Cheese, feta	small matchbox-size piece	2.5	
Cheese, Cheddar type, half fat	small matchbox-size piece	3	
Cheese, Mozzarella, fresh	small matchbox-size piece	3	
Cheese, Brie	small matchbox-size piece	3.5	
Cheese, Cheshire	small matchbox-size piece	4	

Food	Portion Size	GISs	Special Comments
Cheese, Swiss	small matchbox-size piece	4	
Cheese, Cheddar	small matchbox-size piece	4.5	grated goes further, use 3 tablespoons
Cheese, Stilton, blue	small matchbox-size piece	4.5	

NUTS (use nuts in cooking to provide protein)

Food	Portion Size	GISs	Special Comments
Peanuts, dry roasted	small pack (1 oz)	3	high in fat but low in saturates and GI, choose nuts once a day strictly in these amounts
Peanuts, roasted and salted	small pack (1 oz)	3	high in fat but low in saturates and GI, choose nuts once a day strictly in these amounts
Walnuts	6 halves	3	throw them into salad; choose nuts once a day strictly in these amounts
Almonds	10–12 almonds	3	high in fat but low in GI and saturates, choose once a day strictly in these amounts
Cashew nuts	15 cashews	3.5	high in fat but low in GI, choose nuts once a day strictly in these amounts

VEGETABLES
(packed with free choices)

Food	Portion Size	GISs
Alfalfa sprouts	as desired	0
Artichoke, globe	as desired	0
Asparagus	as desired	0
Asparagus, canned, drained	as desired	0
Bamboo shoots, canned, drained	as desired	0
Broccoli, green, frozen, steamed	as desired	0
Broccoli, green, raw	as desired	0
Broccoli, green, steamed	as desired	0
Broccoli, purple sprouting, steamed	as desired	0

Food	Portion Size	GISs	Special Comments
Cabbage, spring, steamed	as desired	0	
Cabbage, winter, steamed	as desired	0	
Cabbage, Chinese, raw	as desired	0	
Cabbage, frozen, steamed	as desired	0	
Cabbage, red, steamed	as desired	0	
Cabbage, Savoy, steamed	as desired	0	
Cabbage, summer, steamed	as desired	0	
Cabbage, white, steamed	as desired	0	
Cauliflower, frozen, steamed	as desired	0	
Cauliflower, raw	as desired	0	
Cauliflower, steamed	as desired	0	
Celeriac, raw	as desired	0	
Celeriac, steamed	as desired	0	
Celery, raw	as desired	0	
Celery, steamed	as desired	0	
Chard, Swiss, raw	as desired	0	
Chard, Swiss, steamed	as desired	0	
Chicory, raw	as desired	0	
Chicory, steamed	as desired	0	
Corn, baby, canned, drained	as desired	0	
Corn, baby, fresh and frozen, steamed	as desired	0	
Cucumber, raw	as desired	0	
Curly kale, steamed	as desired	0	
Eggplant, grilled	as desired	0	
Endive, raw	as desired	0	
Fennel, raw	as desired	0	
Fennel, steamed	as desired	0	
Grape leaves, preserved in brine	as desired	0	
Leeks, steamed	as desired	0	
Lettuce, butter, raw	as desired	0	
Lettuce, Iceberg, raw	as desired	0	
Lettuce, mixed leaves	as desired	0	

Food	Portion Size	GISs	Special Comments
Mushrooms, raw	as desired	0	
Mushrooms, canned, drained	as desired	0	
Mushrooms, oyster, raw	as desired	0	
Mushrooms, steamed	as desired	0	
Mushrooms, straw, canned, drained	as desired	0	
Mustard leaves, steamed	as desired	0	
Okra, canned, drained	as desired	0	
Okra, steamed	as desired	0	
Onions, cooked	as desired	0	
Onions, pickled, cocktail/ silverskin, drained	as desired	0	
Peppers, steamed	as desired	0	
Peppers, raw	as desired	0	
Raddiccio, raw	as desired	0	
Radish, red, raw	as desired	0	
Radish, white/mooli, raw	as desired	0	
Sauerkraut	as desired	0	
Shallots, raw	as desired	0	
Spinach, canned, drained	as desired	0	
Spinach, frozen, steamed	as desired	0	
Spinach, raw	as desired	0	
Spinach, steamed	as desired	0	
Spring onions, bulbs and tops, raw	as desired	0	
Tomatoes, canned, with juice	as desired	0	
Tomatoes, cherry, raw	as desired	0	
Tomatoes, raw	as desired	0	
Turnip, steamed	as desired	0	
Watercress, raw	as desired	0	
Yellow squash, steamed	as desired	0	
Zucchini, raw	as desired	0	
Zucchini, steamed	as desired	0	
Brussels sprouts, frozen, steamed	12 sprouts	0.5	
Brussels sprouts, steamed	12 sprouts	0.5	

Food	Portion Size	GISs	Special Comments
Carrot, average raw	1 large carrot	0.5	GI is high but it has few carbs and won't spike up blood sugar so GIS is low
Carrots, fresh, steamed	2 tablespoons	0.5	
Carrots, frozen, steamed	2 tablespoons	0.5	
Carrots, young, steamed	2 tablespoons	0.5	
Zucchini, sautéed	1 zucchini	1	use spray oil
Navy beans, dried, steamed	5 oz	1	
Butter beans, dried, boiled	5 oz	1.5	
Plantain, steamed	1 plantain	1.5	
Seaweed, nori, dried, raw	2 tablespoons	1.5	contains the antioxidant selenium
Yam, baked	medium size	1.5	
Yam, boiled	medium size	1.5	
Yam, steamed	medium size	1.5	
Beets, pickled, drained	4 slices	2	
Mushrooms, common, stir-fried	2 tablespoons	2	or use a little spray oil and count as 0 GISs
Peas, fresh, steamed	3 tablespoons	2	
Peas, frozen, steamed	3 tablespoons	2	
Corn, on-the-cob, whole, steamed	1 cob	2	
Corn, kernels, canned,	3 tablespoons	2.5	choose canned veggies in in drained, unsalted, unsweetened water
Corn, kernels, fresh, cooked	3 tablespoons	2.5	
Beets, cooked	4 slices	2.5	
New potatoes, boiled	4 new potatoes	3	keep skins on
New potatoes, canned, drained	4 new potatoes	3	
Potatoes, boiled	3 egg-size potatoes	3	
Pumpkin, cooked	2 slices	3	
Rutabaga, steamed	2 tablespoons	3	
Sweet potato, boiled	1 small potato	3	
Sweet potato, steamed	1 small potato	3	
Sweet potato, baked	1 small potato	3.5	
Fava beans, boiled	2 tablespoons	3.5	

Food	Portion Size	GISs	Special Comments
French fries, straight cut, frozen, oven baked	6 tablespoons	5	choose 5% fat versions
French fries, fast food outlet	2 serving spoons	6	
Instant mashed potato made with water	2 scoops	7	use the same GIS for home-made, add any GISs from milk or butter
Potatoes, baked	1 medium potato	7	add a low GIS carb
Parsnip, steamed	2 tablespoons	7	a great veggie, but high in GI
Parsnip, roast	2 tablespoons	7.5	

FRUIT

(fruit gets the gold star)

Grapefruit	1 grapefruit	0	rich in potassium which helps to regulate blood pressure
Strawberries	5 oz	0	keep to portion size if you want to have them GIS-free
Apples	1 apple	0.5	the whole fruit has all the fiber, choose it over fruit juice
Cherries	12 cherries	0.5	
Olives	10 olives	0.5	olives with pits take longer to eat so you might eat less
Peaches, canned in juice	6 slices	0.5	
Pears	1 pear	0.5	
Plums	3 plums	0.5	
Fruit cocktail, canned in juice	½ large can	1	
Kiwi	2 kiwi	1.5	abundant in vitamin C
Oranges	1 large orange	1.5	
Peaches	1 peach	1.5	
Pears, canned in juice	2 pear halves	1.5	
Prunes, ready-to-eat	8 prunes	1.5	
Watermelon	1 slice	3.5	GI is high, but it has few carbs and will not spike up blood sugar so GI value is low

Food	Portion Size	GISs	Special Comments
Apricots, dried	6 apricots	2	good source of fiber and beta-carotene
Avocado	1 small	2	
Bananas	1 small banana	2	great source of potassium
Cantaloupe	½ melon	2	
Dates, dried	4 dates	2	
Grapes, red or green	15 grapes	2	
Mango	1 small mango	2	
Apricots, fresh	3 apricots	2.5	
Pineapple	1 slice	2.5	
Figs, dried	2 figs	3	
Raisins	2 handfuls	3	
Golden raisins	2 handfuls	3	

DRINKS

Food	Portion Size	GISs	Special Comments
Diet soft drinks	as desired	0	you could go for decaf versions
Water, sparkling	as desired	0	
Water, still	as desired	0	
Water, sugar-free flavored	as desired	0	check no added sugar
Tomato juice	5 oz	0	add some Worcester sauce for zing!
Apple juice, unsweetened	5 oz	1.5	cloudy has a slightly lower GI
Grapefruit juice, unsweetened	5 oz	1.5	
Orange juice, unsweetened	5 oz	1.5	
Pineapple juice, unsweetened	5 oz	1.5	
Cranberry juice	5 oz	3	diet versions are lower in calories, but GI value is not available
Coffee, no sugar	as desired	0	use milk from allowance
Tea, no sugar	as desired	0	use milk from allowance

Food	Portion Size	GISs	Special Comments

CRACKERS AND SNACKS

(nuts in shells take longer to eat, so you may end up having less)

Food	Portion Size	GISs	Special Comments
Crispbread, rye	2 crispbread	3	
Ryvita	2 crispbread	3	
Whole wheat crackers	2 crackers	3	
Stoned Wheat Thins	2 crackers	3	
Oat cakes	2 oat cakes	3.5	use the same GIS for oatmeal biscuits
Melba toast, plain	2 toast	7	
Rice cakes	2 cakes	7	calories per rice cake are low, but GI is high
Sesame seeds	2 teaspoons	1	throw them into GIS-free salad for extra crunch
Peanuts, dry roasted	small pack (1 oz)	3	high in fat but low in GI and saturates, choose nuts once a day strictly in these amounts
Peanuts, roasted and salted	small pack (1 oz)	3	high in fat but low in GI and saturates, choose nuts once a day strictly in these amounts
Walnuts	6 halves	3	high in fat but low in GI and saturates, choose nuts once a day strictly in these amounts
Almonds	10–12 almonds	3	high in fat but low in GI and saturates, choose nuts once a day strictly in these amounts
Cashew nuts	15 cashews	3.5	high in fat but low in GI, choose nuts once a day strictly in these amounts
Popcorn, plain, popped	5 tablespoons	4	choose lower-fat varieties, high GI, see recipe for Chili Peanut Popcorn page 131
Chewy granola and dried fruit bar	45-50 gram bar	4.5	
Crunchy granola and dried fruit bar	45–50 gram bar	4.5	
Pretzels	1 oz	6	low-fat snack but high in GI

Food	Portion Size	GISs	Special Comments

SEASONINGS
(choose as often as you like)

Food	Portion Size	GISs	Special Comments
Chili sauce		0	
Mustard		0	
Soy sauce		0	try low-sodium types
Worcestershire sauce		0	
Vinegar (rice, balsamic, malt, wine)		0	
Oil, spray oil		0	5 sprays per dish, strict portion limit
Dressing, fat-free		0	
Artificial sweeteners		0	
Jell-O, sugar-free		0	
Jelly, sugar-free		0	
Stock cube		0	try low-sodium types
Tomato purée		0	
Herbs, fresh or dried		0	
Spices, fresh (e.g. garlic, ginger, chili)		0	
Spices, ground (e.g. paprika, chili powder, curry powder)		0	
Spices, whole (e.g. cumin seeds, coriander seeds, caraway seeds)		0	
Salt		0	keep added salt to a minimum
Salt substitutes		0	
Pepper		0	

FATTY AND SUGARY FOODS
(keep to a minimum)

PASTRY

Food	Portion Size	GISs	Special Comments
Banana bread	1 slice	4.5	
Muffins, chocolate chip	1 muffin	5	choosing a smaller one means less fat
Muffins, blueberry	1 muffin	5	

Food	Portion Size	GISs	Special Comments
Muffins, oat bran	1 muffin	5	
Pound cake, Sara Lee	1 slice	5	
Danish pastries	small pastry	5.5	
Sponge cake	small slice	6	watch portion size
Croissants	1 croissant	6	
Waffles	1 waffle	6.5	
Doughnuts, plain	1 doughnut	7.5	
Shortbread	2 cookies	7.5	
Scone, plain	1 scone	10	very high GI, hence high GIS value

FATS AND OILS (opt for monounsaturated ones)

Food	Portion Size	GISs	Special Comments
Spread, low-fat	scraping	0.5	
Spread, half fat, unsaturated	scraping	0.5	some are mono-unsaturated
Spread, very low-fat, unsaturated	1 teaspoon	0.5	
Butter	scraping	1	
Spread, low-fat	1 teaspoon	1	
Spread, half fat, unsaturated	1 teaspoon	1	
Oil, olive oil	1 teaspoon	1.5	monounsaturated
Oil, rapeseed oil	1 teaspoon	1.5	monounsaturated. Also sometimes sold as vegetable oil—check label
Butter	1 teaspoon	2	
Oil, sunflower oil	1 teaspoon	2	if cooking for 4, use 4 tsp and then count your portion as 2 GISs
Oil, vegetable oil, mixed	1 teaspoon	2	

FAST FOOD AND PROCESSED FOODS

Food	Portion Size	GISs	Special Comments
Instant gravy	2 serving spoons	0.5	can be high in salt, but lower in fat than using meat juices
Ravioli, meat	12 ravioli	1.5	

Food	Portion Size	GISs	Special Comments
Sushi	6 small pieces	2.5	
Wheat tortilla with refried pinto beans and tomato sauce	1 tortilla ½ cup beans 1 tbsp sauce	2.5	
Tortellini, cheese	12 tortellini	3	remember to add any GISs from sauces
Grape leaves, stuffed with rice	8 medium leaves	3	
Bacon, back, grilled	3 slices	3	GI of turkey slices is not available, but they are a lower-fat choice
Beef sausages, grilled is	2 sausages	3	GI of lower-fat sausages not available, but they are a better choice
Pork sausages, grilled	2 sausages	3	
Bacon, middle, grilled	3 slices	3.5	
Burgers, chilled/frozen, grilled	2 burgers	3.5	
Pizza, cheese and tomato, deep dish	2 slices from medium (9" diameter) or 1 slice of large (12" diameter)	3.5	GI of other pizza toppings not available—if choosing meat toppings, opt for lower-fat types
Pizza, cheese and tomato, thin crust	2 slices from medium (9" diameter) or 1 slice of large (12" diameter)	3.5	GI of other pizza toppings not available—avoid extra cheese
Pizza, vegetarian	2 slices from medium (9" diameter) or 1 slice of large (12" diameter)	3.5	choose less cheese and more veggies
Chicken nuggets, take-out	6 nuggets	4	
Macaroni and cheese	6 tablespoons	4	tomato-based sauces tend to be lower in calories and richer in antioxidants
Chicken, stir-fried with rice and vegetables, frozen	pre-packaged meal	4.5	
French fries, straight cut, frozen, oven baked	6 tablespoons	5	
French fries, fast food outlet	6 tablespoons	6	

Food	Portion Size	GISs	Special Comments
Taco shells, baked	1 shell	7	

CHIPS

Food	Portion Size	GISs	Special Comments
Corn chips	small bag (30 g)	6	
Potato chips	small bag (25 g)	6.5	

SUGARY FOODS

Food	Portion Size	GISs	Special Comments
Jam, reduced sugar	1 teaspoon	0.5	
Fructose	2 teaspoons	1	
Honey	1 teaspoon	1	
Jam	1 teaspoon	1	
Marmalade	1 teaspoon	1	
Milk chocolate	1 square piece	1.5	
Milk chocolate	1 treat-size bar (15 g)	2	
Snickers® bar	1 fun size (19 g)	2	
Ice cream, reduced calorie	2 scoops	2.5	
Sugar	2 teaspoons	2.5	
Twix®	1 mini Twix® (21 g)	2.5	
Mars® bar	1 fun size (19 g)	3	
Ice cream, vanilla	2 scoops	4	
Jellybeans	6 jelly beans	4	
Nougat	4 pieces	4	
Chocolate-covered peanuts (e.g. M&M'S®)	1 small pack (2 oz)	5	

Food	Portion Size	GISs	Special Comments

ALPHABETICAL GIS TABLE

BEANS AND LENTILS *all beans and lentils count once a day as one of your five fruit and vegetables. These are also protein foods and if you choose them as your protein, then choose another carb.*

FATS AND OILS *opt for monounsaturated ones and keep to a minimum*

FRUIT *have five fruit and vegetables a day, they're rich in antioxidants*

FISH *choose fish twice a week, one should be oily fish which is rich in omega-3 fats*

NUTS *nuts in shells take longer to eat, which may help you have less when snacking*

PASTA *add GISs from sauces. Use 2 oz raw per portion*

RICE AND GRAINS *keep rice grains whole rather than soft and mushy*

VEGETABLES *some of these are part of meal carbs since they are high in starch*

A

Food	Portion Size	GISs	Special Comments
Alfalfa sprouts	as desired	0	
Apples	1 apple	0.5	the whole fruit has all the fiber, choose it over fruit juice
Apricots, dried	6 apricots	2	good source of fiber and beta-carotene
Apricots, fresh	3 apricots	2.5	
Artichoke, globe	as desired	0	
Artificial sweeteners	as desired	0	
Asparagus	as desired	0	
Asparagus, canned, drained	as desired	0	
Avocado	1 small	2	

B

Food	Portion Size	GISs	Special Comments
Bacon, back, grilled	3 slices	3	GI of turkey bacon is not available, but they are a lower-fat choice
Bacon, middle, grilled	3 slices	3.5	
Beans, baked, canned in tomato sauce	5 oz	2	low in GI, high in versatility

Food	Portion Size	GISs	Special Comments
Bamboo shoots, canned, drained	as desired	0	
Banana bread	1 slice	4.5	
Bananas	1 small banana	2	great source of potassium
Barley, pearl, cooked	5 oz	1.5	throw some into soups and stews
Beans, broad, canned	7 oz	4	
Beans, broad, dried, cooked	5 oz	3.5	
Beans, broad, frozen, cooked	5 oz	4	
Beans, butter beans, dried, cooked	5 oz	1.5	
Beans, chili, canned	7 oz	1	
Beans, navy, dried, cooked	5 oz	1	
Beans, navy, dried, steamed	5 oz	1	
Beans, mung, whole, dried, cooked	5 oz	2	
Beans, pinto, dried, cooked	5 oz	1.5	
Beans, red kidney, canned	7 oz	2	
Beans, red kidney, dried, cooked	5 oz	1.5	you can use a combination of beans in smaller portions for the same GISs
Beef sausages, grilled	2 sausages	3	GI of lower-fat sausages is not available, but they are a better choice
Beef, sirloin joint, roasted, lean	3 slices	2	
Beef stew, made with lean beef	6 tablespoons	1.5	limit or avoid fat in cooking
Beef, ground, stewed	6 tablespoons	2.5	choose lean beef
Beef, rump steak, lean, grilled	5 oz steak	2	cooked weight
Beef, topside, roasted well-done, lean	3 slices	2.5	
Beets, cooked	4 slices	2.5	
Beets, pickled, drained	4 slices	2	
Black-eyed peas, dried, cooked	5 oz	1.5	
Bread, bagels, plain	1 bagel	6	a low-GIS carb filling (e.g. vegetables) helps to reduce the GI of the meal
Bread, baguette	1 individual	9	a great food but a very high GI. Eat always with a

Food	Portion Size	GISs	Special Comments
			low-GIS carb filling (e.g. corn)
Bread, barley	2 slices	3	
Bread, barley and sunflower	2 slices	4.5	
Bread, hamburger buns	1 bun	5	
Bread, Melba toast, plain	2 toasts	7	
Bread, mixed grain	2 slices	3.5	wholegrains are richer in B vitamins than refined grains
Bread, pita	1 pita	5	whole wheat ones are higher in fiber
Bread, pumpernickel	2 slices	3.5	
Bread, rye	2 slices	4.5	
Bread, white	2 slices	5.5	
Bread, white, with added fiber	2 slices	4.5	
Bread, whole wheat	2 slices	5.5	opt for stoneground as it is more coarse and thus has a lower GI
Breakfast cereals			*see Cereal*
Broccoli, green, frozen, steamed	as desired	0	
Broccoli, green, raw	as desired	0	
Broccoli, green, steamed	as desired	0	
Broccoli, purple sprouting, steamed	as desired	0	
Brussels sprouts, frozen, steamed	12 sprouts	0.5	
Brussels sprouts, steamed	12 sprouts	0.5	
Bulgur wheat, cooked	5 oz	2	
Butter	scraping	1	
Butter	1 teaspoon	2	

C

Cabbage, spring, steamed	as desired	0	
Cabbage, winter, steamed	as desired	0	
Cabbage, Chinese, raw	as desired	0	
Cabbage, frozen, steamed	as desired	0	

Food	Portion Size	GISs	Special Comments
Cabbage, red, steamed	as desired	0	
Cabbage, Savoy, steamed	as desired	0	
Cabbage, summer, steamed	as desired	0	
Cabbage, white, steamed	as desired	0	
Cantaloupe	½ melon	2	
Carrot, average, raw	1 large carrot	0.5	GI is high, but it has few carbs and won't spike up blood sugar so GIS is low
Carrots, fresh, steamed	2 tablespoons	0.5	
Carrots, frozen, steamed	2 tablespoons	0.5	
Carrots, young, steamed	2 tablespoons	0.5	
Cauliflower, frozen, steamed	as desired	0	
Cauliflower, raw	as desired	0	
Cauliflower, steamed	as desired	0	
Celeriac, raw	as desired	0	
Celeriac, steamed	as desired	0	
Celery, raw	as desired	0	
Celery, steamed	as desired	0	
Cereal, All Bran and 2% milk	5 tablespoons+ 7 oz	2	try it with sliced banana
Cereal, Bran Flakes and 2% milk`	4 tablespoons+ 7 oz	4	
Cereal, Cornflakes and 2% milk	5 tablespoons+ 7 oz	4.5	
Cereal, Grapenuts and 2% milk	5 tablespoons+ 7 oz	4.5	
Cereal, muesli and 2% milk	3 tablespoons+ 7 oz	4	
Cereal, muesli, reduced sugar and 2% milk	3 tablespoons+ 7 oz	4	
Cereal, muesli, Swiss-style, and 2% milk	3 tablespoons+ 7 oz	4	
Cereal, Nutrigrain and 2% milk	5 tablespoons+ 7 oz	4.5	
Cereal, Puffed Wheat and 2% milk	5 tablespoons+ 7 oz	4	

Food	Portion Size	GISs	Special Comments
Cereal, Rice Krispies and 2% milk	7 tablespoons+ 7 oz	5.5	
Cereal, Shredded Wheat and 2% milk	2 biscuits+ 7 oz	4.5	
Cereal, Special K and 2% milk	5 tablespoons+ 7 oz	4	
Cereal, Raisin Bran and 2% milk	4 tablespoons+ 7 oz	4.5	
Chard, Swiss, raw	as desired	0	
Chard, Swiss, steamed	as desired	0	
Cheese, Brie	small matchbox-size piece	3.5	
Cheese, Cheddar	small matchbox-size piece	4.5	grated goes further, use 3 tablespoons
Cheese, Cheddar type, half fat	small matchbox-size piece	3	
Cheese, cottage cheese, plain	5 oz	1.5	
Cheese, cottage cheese, plain, reduced-fat	5 oz	1	
Cheese, Swiss	small matchbox-size piece	4	
Cheese, feta	small matchbox-size piece	2.5	
Cheese, mozzarella, fresh	small matchbox-size piece	3	
Cheese, ricotta	small tub (5 oz)	1.5	
Cheese, Stilton, blue	small matchbox-size piece	4.5	
Cherries	12 cherries	0.5	
Chickpeas, canned	7 oz	2	great spiced up as a snack – add chili sauce
Chickpeas, split, dried, cooked	5 oz	2.5	
Chickpeas, whole, dried, cooked	5 oz	1.5	
Chicken nuggets, takeout	6 nuggets	4	
Chicken, breast chunks or strips	6 tablespoons	2	
Chicken, breast, skinless, roasted	1 medium	2	
Chicken, drumstick, skinless, roasted	2 drumsticks	2	chicken breast is lower in fat

Food	Portion Size	GISs	Special Comments
Chicken, leg, skinless, roasted	1 medium	2	
Chicken, roasted	3 slices	2	avoid the skin, breast pieces are lower in fat
Chicken, stir-fried with rice and vegetables, frozen	packaged serving	4.5	
Chicken, thigh, skinless, roasted	1 medium	2	
Chicken, wing, skinless, roasted	4 wings	2	see recipe page 127
Chicory, raw	as desired	0	
Chicory, steamed	as desired	0	
Chili sauce	as desired	0	
Chocolate-covered peanuts (e.g. M&M'S®)	1 small pack (47 g)	5	
Cod, baked	1 filet	1	
Cod, grilled	1 filet	1	
Coffee	as desired	0	use milk from allowance
Cookies, shortbread	2 pieces	7.5	
Corn, baby, canned, drained	as desired	0	
Corn, baby, fresh and frozen, steamed	as desired	0	
Corn, kernels, canned,	3 tablespoons	2.5	choose drained unsalted, unsweetened water
Corn, kernels, fresh, cooked	3 tablespoons	2.5	
Corn, on-the-cob, whole, steamed	1 cob	2	
Corn chips	small packet (30 g)	6	
Corned beef, canned	2 slices	2.5	watch the salt!
Couscous, cooked	5 oz	3.5	a nice change from rice
Crab	2 tablespoons crab meat	1.5	
Crackers, crispbread, rye	2 crackers	3	
Crackers, Ryvita	2 crispbreads	3	
Crackers, Stoned Wheat Thins	2 crackers	3	
Crackers, whole wheat	2 crackers	3	
Croissants	1 croissant	6	
Cucumber, raw	as desired	0	
Curly kale, steamed	as desired	0	

Food	Portion Size	GISs	Special Comments
D			
Danish pastries	small pastry	5.5	
Dates, dried	4 dates	2	
Diet soft drinks	as desired	0	you could go for decaf versions
Doughnuts	1 doughnut	7.5	
Dressing, fat-free	as desired	0	avoid added sugar
Drinkable yogurt	7 oz if available	1	choose reduced calorie
Duck, roasted	3 slices	2	avoid the skin
E			
Eggs, boiled	2 eggs	1.5	
Eggs, fried	2 eggs	3	
Eggs, poached	2 eggs	1.5	
Eggs, scrambled, with milk and 1 tsp oil	2 eggs	3	
Eggplant, grilled	as desired	0	
Endive, raw	as desired	0	
F			
Fennel, raw	as desired	0	
Fennel, steamed	as desired	0	
Figs, dried	2 figs	3	
Fish sticks, cod, grilled	4 sticks	2	
Flounder, steamed or grilled	1 filet	1	
French fries, fast food outlet	6 tablespoons	6	
French fries, straight cut, frozen, oven baked	6 tablespoons	5	choose 5% fat varieties
Fructose	2 teaspoons	1	
Fruit cocktail, canned in juice	7 oz	1	
G			
Gherkins, pickled, drained	as desired	0	
Granola and dried fruit bar chewy	45–50 gram bar	4.5	

Food	Portion Size	GISs	Special Comments
Granola and dried fruit bar, crunchy	45–50 gram bar	4.5	
Grape leaves, preserved in brine	as desired	0	
Grape leaves, stuffed with rice	8 medium vine leaves	3	
Grapefruit	1 grapefruit	0	rich in potassium which helps to regulate blood pressure
Grapefruit juice, unsweetened	1 glass (5 oz)	1.5	
Grapes	15 grapes	2	
Gravy, instant	6 tablespoons	0.5	can be high in salt, but lower in fat than using meat juices

H

Food	Portion Size	GISs	Special Comments
Haddock, smoked	1 filet	1.5	smoked foods are higher in salt, so limit amounts
Haddock, steamed or grilled	1 filet	1	
Halibut, steamed or grilled	1 filet	1.5	
Ham	2 slices	1.5	
Hamburgers, chilled/frozen, grilled	2 hamburgers	3.5	
Herbs, fresh or dried	as desired	0	
Herring, grilled	2 filets	2	a source of healthy omega-3 fats
Honey	1 teaspoon	1	

I

Food	Portion Size	GISs	Special Comments
Ice cream, reduced calorie	2 scoops	2.5	
Ice cream, vanilla	2 scoops	4	

J

Food	Portion Size	GISs	Special Comments
Jam	1 teaspoon	1	
Jam, reduced sugar	1 teaspoon	0.5	
Jell-O, sugar-free	as desired	0	
Jelly, sugar-free	as desired	0	
Jellybeans	6 jelly beans	4	
Juice, apple, unsweetened	1 glass (5 oz)	1.5	cloudy has a slightly lower GI

Food	Portion Size	GISs	Special Comments
Juice, cranberry	1 glass (5 oz)	3	diet versions are lower in calories, but GI value is not available
Juice, grapefruit, unsweetened	1 glass (5 oz)	1.5	
Juice, orange, unsweetened	1 glass (5 oz))	1.5	
Juice, pineapple, unsweetened	1 glass (5 oz)	1.5	
Juice, tomato	1 glass (5 oz)	0	add some Worcester sauce for zing!

K

Food	Portion Size	GISs	Special Comments
Kidney, lamb, sautéed	2 kidneys	2	
Kiwi fruit	2 kiwi	1.5	abundant in vitamin C

L

Food	Portion Size	GISs	Special Comments
Lamb, loin chops, grilled, lean	2 chops	1.5	
Leeks, steamed	as desired	0	
Lemon sole, steamed or grilled	1 filet	1	
Lentils, black gram, urad gram, dried, cooked	5 oz	2	
Lentils, red, split, dried, cooked	5 oz	1	
Lettuce, butter, raw	as desired	0	
Lettuce, Iceberg, raw	as desired	0	
Lettuce, mixed leaves	as desired	0	
Liver sausage	1 slice	2.5	all sausages tend to be high in salt and very processed
Liver, lamb, sautéed	2 slices	2.5	rich in iron, great for the immune system
Liver, ox, stewed	3 tablespoons	2	rich in iron and vitamin B12
Lobster	2 tablespoons	1.5	

M

Food	Portion Size	GISs	Special Comments
Macaroni and cheese	6 tablespoons	4	tomato-based sauces tend to be lower in calories and richer in

Food	Portion Size	GISs	Special Comments
			antioxidants
Mackerel, canned in brine, drained	small can	2.5	a source of healthy omega-3 fats
Mangoes	1 small mango	2	
Marmalade	1 teaspoon	1	
Mars® bar	1 fun size (19 g)	3	
Milk, 2%	7 oz	0.5	
Milk, skim	7 oz	0.5	
Milk chocolate	1 square piece	1.5	
Milk chocolate	1 treat-sized bar (15g)	2	
Muffins, chocolate chip	1 muffin	5	choosing a smaller one means less fat
Muffins, blueberry	1 muffin	5	
Muffins, oat bran	1 muffin	5	
Mushrooms, raw	as desired	0	
Mushrooms, canned, drained	as desired	0	
Mushrooms, common, stir-fried	2 tablespoons	2	use 5 sprays instead of oil and count as 0
Mushrooms, oyster, raw	as desired	0	
Mushrooms, steamed	as desired	0	
Mushrooms, straw, canned, drained	as desired	0	
Mussels	6 mussels	1.5	
Mustard	as desired	0	
Mustard leaves, steamed	as desired	0	

N

Food	Portion Size	GISs	Special Comments
Nougat	4 pieces	4	
Nuts, almonds	10–12 almonds	3	high in fat but low in GI and saturates, choose nuts once a day strictly in these amounts
Nuts, cashews	15 cashews	3.5	high in fat but low in GI, choose nuts once a day strictly in these amounts

Food	Portion Size	GISs	Special Comments
Nuts, peanuts, dry roasted	1 oz 1 oz	3	high in fat but low in GI and saturates, choose nuts once a day strictly in these amounts
Nuts, peanuts, roasted and salted	1 oz	3	high in fat but low in GI and saturates, choose nuts once a day strictly in these amounts
Nuts, walnuts	6 halves	3	high in fat but low in saturates and GI, choose nuts once a day strictly in these amounts

O

Food	Portion Size	GISs	Special Comments
Oat cakes	2 oat cakes	3.5	use the same GIS for oatmeal biscuits
Oatmeal, instant made with 2% milk	follow pack instructions using 7 oz	4.5	a package at work could be a convenient breakfast
Oatmeal, made with milk and water	6 tablespoons of made-up oatmeal using 3 oz milk and water as required	3.5	you could try skim milk, 7 oz, instead Use a little sweetener, honey or fructose if you like, add the GISs
Oatmeal, made with water	8 tablespoons of made-up oatmeal as per pack instructions	3	
Oil, olive oil	1 teaspoon	1.5	monounsaturated
Oil, rapeseed oil	1 teaspoon	1.5	monounsaturated. Also sometimes sold as vegetable oil —check label
Oil, spray oil	5 sprays per dish	0	strict portion limit
Oil, sunflower oil	1 teaspoon	2	if cooking for 4, use 4 teaspoons and then count your portion as 2 GISs
Oil, vegetable oil, mixed	1 teaspoon	2	
Okra, canned, drained	as desired	0	
Okra, steamed	as desired	0	
Olives	10 olives	0.5	olives with pits take longer to eat so you eat less!

Food	Portion Size	GISs	Special Comments
Omelette, plain, made with 1 tsp oil	2 eggs	3	
Onions, cooked	as desired	0	
Onions, pickled, cocktail/silverskin, drained	as desired	0	
Oranges	1 large orange	1.5	
Oysters	1 dozen oysters	1	shellfish are a good source of zinc, great for immune function

P

Food	Portion Size	GISs	Special Comments
Parsnip, boiled	2 tablespoons	7	serve with low-GIS vegetables
Parsnip, roast	2 tablespoons	7.5	
Parsnip, steamed	2 tablespoons	7	a great vegetable, but high in GI
Pasta, fettucine, egg, cooked	5 tablespoons	1.5	
Pasta, linguini, thick, cooked	5 tablespoons	2.5	
Pasta, linguini, thin, cooked	5 tablespoons	2.5	
Pasta, macaroni, cooked	5 tablespoons	2	
Pasta, noodles, instant, cooked	5 tablespoons	2	
Pasta, noodles, rice, cooked	5 tablespoons	3	
Pasta, plain, cooked	5 tablespoons	3	
Pasta, ravioli, meat	12 ravioli	1.5	
Pasta, spaghetti, white, cooked	5 tablespoons	1.5	use 2 oz raw
Pasta, spaghetti, whole wheat, cooked	5 tablespoons	1.5	
Pasta, tortellini, cheese	12 tortellini	3	remember to add any GISs from sauces
Peaches	1 peach	1.5	
Peaches, canned in juice	6 slices	0.5	
Pears	1 pear	0.5	
Pears, canned in juice	2 pear halves	1.5	
Peas, fresh, steamed	3 tablespoons	2	
Pepper, whole or ground	as desired	0	
Peppers, steamed	as desired	0	
Peppers, raw	as desired	0	

Food	Portion Size	GISs	Special Comments
Pigeon peas, whole, dried, cooked	5 oz	1.5	
Pineapple	1 slice	2.5	
Pineapple juice, unsweetened	1 glass (5 oz)	1.5	
Pizza, cheese and tomato, deep dish	2 slices from medium (9" diameter) or 1 slice of large (12" diameter)	3.5	GI of other pizza toppings not available—avoid extra cheese
Pizza, cheese and tomato, thin crust	2 slices from medium (9" diameter) or 1 slice of large (12" diameter)	3.5	GI of other pizza toppings not available—if choosing meat toppings, opt for lower-fat types
Pizza, vegetarian	2 slices from medium (9" diameter) or 1 slice of large (12" diameter)	3.5	choose less cheese and more veggies
Plantain, boiled	1 plantain	1.5	available from West Indian shops
Plantain, steamed	1 plantain	1.5	
Plums	3 plums	0.5	
Popcorn, plain	5 tablespoons	4	choose lower-fat varieties high GI
Pork, leg joint, roasted	3 slices	2	
Pork sausages, grilled	2 sausages	3	
Pork, loin chops, grilled, lean	1 chop	2	
Potato chips	small bag (25 g)	6.5	
Potato, instant mashed, made with water	2 scoops	7	use the same GIS for home-made, add any GISs from milk or butter
Potatoes, new, boiled	4 new potatoes	3	
Potatoes, new, canned, drained	4 new potatoes	3	
Potatoes, baked	1 medium potato	7	serve with a low-GIS carb such as baked beans and salad
Potatoes, boiled	3 egg-size potatoes	3	

Food	Portion Size	GISs	Special Comments
Pound cake, Sara Lee	1 slice	5	
Pretzels	25 gram portion	6	a low-fat snack but high in GI
Prunes, ready-to-eat	8 prunes	1.5	
Pumpkin, cooked	2 slices	3	

R

Food	Portion Size	GISs	Special Comments
Rabbit, stewed	6 tablespoons	1.5	
Raddiccio, raw	as desired	0	
Radish leaves, raw	as desired	0	
Radish, red, raw	as desired	0	
Radish, white/mooli, raw	as desired	0	
Raisins	2 handfuls	3	
Raisins, golden	2 handfuls	3	
Rice, brown, boiled	6 tablespoons	2.5	
Rice cakes	2 cakes	7	calories per rice cake are low, but GI is high
Rice, white, Bangladeshi, boiled	6 tablespoons	1.5	available from Asian grocers
Rice, white, basmati, boiled	6 tablespoons	2.5	
Rice, white, easy cook, boiled	6 tablespoons	3	
Rice, white, glutinous (sticky), boiled	6 tablespoons	7	
Rice, white, instant, boiled	6 tablespoons	3.5	
Rice, white, jasmine, boiled	6 tablespoons	7.5	
Rice, white, polished, boiled	6 tablespoons	3.5	
Rice, white, precooked, microwaved	6 tablespoons	2.5	
Rice, white, risotto, boiled	6 tablespoons	3.5	
Rutabaga, steamed	2 tablespoons	3	

S

Food	Portion Size	GISs	Special Comments
Salmon, pink, canned in brine, drained	small can	2	a source of healthy omega-3 fats

Food	Portion Size	GISs	Special Comments
Salmon, smoked	3 slices	1.5	a source of healthy omega-3 fats
Salmon, steamed or grilled	1 steak	2	a source of healthy omega-3 fats
Salt	sprinkling	0	keep added salt to a minimum
Salt substitutes	as desired	0	
Sardines, canned in brine, drained	4 sardines	2	a source of healthy omega-3 fats
Sauerkraut	as desired	0	
Scallops, steamed	3 tablespoons	1.5	
Scone, plain	1 scone	10	very high GI, hence high GIS value
Seaweed, nori, dried, raw	2 tablespoons	1.5	contains the antioxidant selenium
Semolina, cooked, dry	5 oz	4.5	
Sesame seeds	2 teaspoons	1	throw them into GIS-free salad for extra crunch
Shallots, raw	as desired	0	
Shrimp	5 oz	1.5	
Shrimp, canned in brine, drained	1 small jar	1	
Snickers® bar	1 fun size (19 g)	2	
Soup, instant noodle	1 soup bowl	2	
Soup, lentil	1 soup bowl	2	
Soup, minestrone, dried, as served	1 soup bowl	0	GI of only these packet soups is available, but you can try other flavors
Soup, tomato, cream of, canned	1 soup bowl	1	
Soup, tomato, dried, as served	1 soup bowl	0.5	
Soy sauce	small amounts	0	try low-sodium types
Soy beans, dried, cooked	5 oz	1.5	GI of some canned beans is not available
Soy yogurt	small jar	2	
Soy milk, unsweetened	7 oz	0.5	soy protein is rich in phytochemicals, shown to reduce blood cholesterol
Spices, fresh (e.g. garlic, ginger,	as desired	0	

Food	Portion Size	GISs	Special Comments
chili)			
Spices, ground (e.g. paprika, chili powder, curry powder)	as desired	0	
Spices, whole (e.g. cumin seeds, coriander seeds, caraway seeds)	as desired	0	
Spinach, canned, drained	as desired	0	
Spinach, frozen, steamed	as desired	0	
Spinach, raw	as desired	0	
Spinach, steamed	as desired	0	
Sponge cake	small slice	6	watch portion size
Spread, half fat, unsaturated	1 teaspoon	1	
Spread, half fat, unsaturated	scraping	0.5	some are mono-unsaturated
Spread, low-fat	scraping	0.5	
Spread, low-fat	1 teaspoon	1	
Spread, very low-fat, unsaturated	1 teaspoon	0.5	
Spring onions, bulbs and tops, raw	as desired	0	
Stock cube	small amounts	0	try low-sodium types
Strawberries	5 oz	0	keep to portion size if you want to have them GIS-free
Sugar	2 teaspoons	2.5	
Sushi	6 mini	2.5	
Sweet potato, baked	1 small potato	3.5	
Sweet potato, boiled	1 small potato	3	
Sweet potato, steamed	1 small potato	3	
Sweet potato, steamed or microwaved	1 small potato	3	

T

Food	Portion Size	GISs	Special Comments
Taco shells, baked	1 shell	7	
Tea	as desired	0	
Tomato purée	as desired	0	
Tomatoes, canned, with juice	as desired	0	make a sauce with onion, garlic and herbs, add to pasta for a low-GIS meal

Food	Portion Size	GISs	Special Comments
Tomatoes, cherry, raw	as desired	0	
Tomatoes, raw	as desired	0	
Tortilla, corn	2 tortillas	3	
Tortilla, wheat	1 wrap	3	
Trout, steamed or grilled	1 fish	1.5	a source of healthy omega-3 fats
Tuna, canned in brine, drained	small can	1	half the calories of canned in oil
Turkey, roasted	2 slices	2	you get three times as much if you use wafer-thin turkey
Turnip, steamed	as desired	0	
Twix®	1 mini Twix®	2.5	

V

Veal, cutlet, sautéed	1 cutlet	2.5	
Veal, fillet, roast	1 filet	2.5	
Vinegar (rice, balsamic, malt, wine)	as desired	0	

W

Waffles	1 waffle	6.5	
Water, sparkling	as desired	0	
Water, still	as desired	0	
Water, sugar-free, flavored	as desired	0	check no added sugar
Watercress, raw	as desired	0	
Watermelon	1 slice	1.5	GI is high, but it has few carbs and will not spike up blood sugar so it gets a low GIS value
Wheat tortilla with refried pinto beans and tomato sauce	1 tortilla, ½ cup beans, 1 tbsp sauce	2.5	
Worcestershire sauce	as desired	0	

Food	Portion Size	GISs	Special Comments
Y			
Yam, baked	medium size	1.5	
Yam, boiled	medium size	1.5	
Yam, steamed	medium size	1.5	
Yellow squash, steamed	as desired	0	
Yogurt, non-fat	5 oz	1	
Yogurt, low-fat, natural	5 oz	1	
Z			
Zucchini, raw	as desired	0	
Zucchini, sauteed	1 zucchini	1	see recipe for GIS-free zucchini boats page 141
Zucchini, steamed	as desired	0	

ATTENTION SCIENCE ADDICTS!

Research, references and further reading

This section is for the real science addicts. It contains summaries of only some of the research on GI and weight loss as well as the published literature that we used as research for this book.

Summary of scientific research

1. Agus MSD, Swain JF, Larson CL, Eckert EA, Ludwig DS (2000). "Dietary composition and physiologic adaptations to energy restriction." *American Journal of Clinical Nutrition* **71**:901–7.

Body weight set point has been suggested as an explanation for poor long-term results of conventional energy-restricted diets in the treatment of obesity. This study aimed to establish if dietary composition affects hormonal and metabolic adaptations to energy restriction. A randomized crossover design was used to compare the effects of a high-GI and a low-GI energy- restricted diet. Ten overweight males were studied for nine days on two separate occasions. The men freely selected foods for the first day and were then randomized to a high-GI energy-restricted diet

(67 percent CHO, 15 percent protein, 18 percent fat) or a low-GI energy-restricted diet (43 percent CHO, 27 percent protein, 30 percent fat). The energy-restricted diets were consumed until day six. On days seven and eight the men remained on the high- or low-Simple GI Diets but were not energy restricted.

The men following the low-GI regime showed a greater level of serum leptin (a hormone that regulates appetite and energy expenditure), a higher resting energy expenditure, lower energy intake from snack foods and a preferential nitrogen balance (an indicator of protein breakdown) to the group who had followed the high-GI regime.

The authors conclude that physiological adaptations to energy restriction can be modified by dietary composition.

2. Bell SJ. Sears B (2003). "Low-Glycemic-load diets: Impact in obesity and chronic diseases." Critical Review in *Food Science and Nutrition* **43**(4): 357–77

This is a review of the data surrounding the public health messages of simple low-fat, high-carbohydrate diets and suggests we should be looking beyond Glycemic Index (GI) and more closely at Glycemic Load (GL). GL reflects the effect of the total day's carbohydrate on insulin secretion and hunger rather than that of individual foods. Foods such as carrots are shown to have a high GI but low GL, and therefore are recommended, while potatoes have a high GI and high GL and should be restricted.

A study at Harvard Medical School randomized 107

obese but otherwise healthy children into a low-GL diet group and a reduced-fat (25–30 percent energy) diet group for four months. The low-GL group lost significantly more weight than the low-fat group with 17 percent of subjects showing a reduction in BMI of 3kg/m^2 .

A 10-year multi-center trial of healthy adults aged 18–39 concluded that a low-GL diet rich in dietary fiber was associated with reduced triglycerides, blood pressure, and LDL cholesterol, and increased HDL cholesterol. Similarly, the Nurses Health Study, which followed 75,521 women aged 38–63 with no history of CVD, concluded that high-fiber dietary GL was directly associated with CVD risk and recommended the classification of carbohydrates by GL.

Both the Nurses Health Study and the Health Professional Follow-up Study looking at 42,759 men showed up to a 40 percent increased risk of developing diabetes in subjects following a high-GL diet to those consuming a low-GL diet. Both of these studies were not exclusively dietary interventions and therefore results may have been influenced by other factors.

Although the authors acknowledge that the current data is mainly from short-term studies, they suggest that public health messages should emphasize the need to incorporate low-GI, low-GL foods into the diet and call for more long-term studies in the future.

3. Ludwig DS (2000). "Dietary glycemic index and obesity." *Journal of Nutrition* **130**:280S–83S.

This review examines the physiological effects of Glycemic Index and argues for the need for controlled clinical trials of a low-Glycemic Index (GI) diet in the treatment of obesity. To date, at least 16 studies have examined the effects of GI on appetite and all but one have demonstrated an increase in satiety, delayed hunger return and reduced food intake following low-GI foods than following high-GI foods. This study compared the effects of three meals of equal energy value comprising either high-GI, medium-GI or low-GI foods. Twelve teenage boys, otherwise healthy with at least 120 percent ideal bodyweight, were evaluated on three separate occasions and randomly fed a test meal as a breakfast and again at lunch. The rapid absorption of glucose from the high-GI breakfast resulted in relatively high insulin and low glycagon concentrations. The same effects applied to test lunches, and subjects consumed significantly more energy after the high-GI lunch than either the medium- or low-GI meals.

While the authors accept there may not be a single optimal diet for the treatment of obesity, they suggest that diets designed to lower insulin response to ingested carbohydrate (for example, low GI) may improve access to stored metabolic fuels. Further, they may decrease hunger and promote weight loss. They go on to describe these diets as containing abundant fruits, vegetables and legumes with moderate amounts of protein and healthful fats and decreased refined carbohydrates and potatoes.

The authors remark on the similarity of the low-Simple

GI Diet with the diet of human ancestors over the last several hundred years.

4. Brand-Miller JC, Holt SHA, Pawlak DB, McMillan J (2002). "Glycemic index and obesity." *American Journal of Clinical Nutrition* **76**:281S–285S.

Although weight loss can be achieved by any means of energy restriction, current dietary guidelines have not prevented weight regain or population-level increases in obesity and overweight. Many high-carbohydrate, low-fat diets may be counterproductive to weight control because they markedly increase postprandial hyperglycemia and hyperinsulinemia. Many high-carbohydrate foods common to Western diets produce a high glycemic response, promoting postprandial carbohydrate oxidation at the expense of fat oxidation, which may promote body-fat increases. In contrast, diets based on low-fat foods that produce a low glycemic response may enhance weight control because they promote satiety, minimize postprandial insulin secretion, and maintain insulin sensitivity.

This hypothesis is supported by several intervention studies in humans in which energy-restricted diets based on low-GI foods produced greater weight loss than equivalent diets based on high-GI foods. Long-term studies in animal models have also shown that diets based on high-GI starches promote weight gain, visceral adiposity, and higher concentrations of fat-metabolizing enzymes than do low-GI starch-controlled diets of equivalent energy value.

In an eight-week study of 12 healthy pregnant women, a high-Simple GI Diet was associated with greater weight at term than was a nutrient-balanced, low-Simple GI Diet. In a study of diet and complications of nearly 3,000 subjects with type 1 diabetes, the GI of the overall diet was an independent predictor of waist circumference in men.

The authors conclude that the findings of this review provide scientific rationale to justify randomized, controlled, multi-center intervention studies comparing the effects of conventional and low-Simple GI Diets on weight control.

5. McManus K, Antinoro L, Sacks F (2001). "A randomized controlled trial of a moderate-fat low-energy diet with a low-fat, low-energy diet for weight loss in overweight adults." *International Journal of Obesity*, **25**, 5: 1503–1511.

Nutrition experts studied 101 overweight men and women, who followed either a moderate-fat diet (35 percent energy from fat), or a standard low-fat diet (20 percent energy from fat). Both groups ate the same total calories (women: 1200 kcal; men: 1500 kcal). The moderate-fat diet encouraged inclusion of good sources of monounsaturated fats such as peanuts, peanut butter, olive oil, rapeseed oil, avocados and other nuts, all foods typically forbidden on standard low-fat diets. Saturated-fat intake was kept low. Subjects could consume peanut butter at breakfast and 1 oz nut snacks each afternoon on the 1200 kcal diet.

Results showed a greater participation rate for those on

the moderate-fat diet that included nuts, with over half sticking to the diet, compared to only one in five sticking to the low-fat diet over the 18-month study period. Both groups lost an average of 11 lb in the first year, although it is the longer-term results that really distinguish the diets. Those following the moderate-fat diet were able to keep off a significant amount of their lost weight, whereas the low-fat group had regained some of their initial weight loss at 18 months. Those on the moderate-fat diet had still managed to keep off a significant amount of weight 2½ years after the start of the study. After 18 months the group which ate 1 oz nuts as part of a healthy diet had reduced their waist size by 2¾ in, whereas the other group had in fact increased theirs by 1 in.

6. Matthias B, Schulze DRPH, Frank B Hu MD (2004). "Dietary approaches to prevent the metabolic syndrome. Quality versus quantity of carbohydrates." *Diabetes Care,* **27**:2.

Prevailing dietary guidelines continue to recommend very high intakes of grain products without a clear distinction between whole and refined grains.* Many popular diets that focus on weight loss, on the other hand, have jumped on the low-carbohydrate bandwagon, prohibiting virtually all carbohydrates, especially in the initial phase of the diet. Both approaches are incompatible with current scientific evidence and can have long-term adverse health implications. **With the growing epidemic of obesity and** the metabolic syndrome, reduction in the consumption of refined carbohydrates and sugar, replaced by minimally processed wholegrain products and healthy sources of fats and protein, should become a major public health priority, together with regular physical activity and weight maintenance.

References and further reading

Food and Agriculture Organization/World Health Organization. Carbohydrates in Human Nutrition. Report of a Joint FAO/WHO Expert Consultation. Rome, 14–18 April 1997. *FAO Food and Nutrition Paper* 66, 1998.

Foster-Powell K, Holt SHA, Brand-Miller JC (2002). "International table of glycemic index and glycemic load values." *American Journal of Clinical Nutrition* **76**:266S–273S.

Jenkins DJA, Kendall CWC, Augustin LSA et al. (2002). "Glycemic index: overview of implications in health and disease." *American Journal of Clinical Nutrition* **76**:266S–273S.

Ludwig DS, Majzoub JA, Al-Zahrani A, Dallal GE, Blanco I, Roberts SB (1999). "High glycemic index foods, overeating, and obesity." *Pediatrics* 103(3).

Jiang R, Manson JE, Stampfer MJ, Liu S, Willett WC, Hu FB

---

* US Department of Agriculture, US Department of Heath and Human Services: *Nutrition and Your Health: Dietary Guidelines for Americans.* Washington, DC, US Government Printing Office, 2000.

(2002). "A prospective study of nut consumption and risk of type 2 diabetes in women." *Journal of the American Medical Association* **288**: 2554–2560.

The New Glucose Revolution (formerly *The GI Factor*), by Dr. Anthony Leeds, Prof. Jennie Brand Miller, Kaye Foster-Powell and Dr. Stephen Colagiuri. Published by Marlow & Company (2002).

FURTHER INFORMATION AND SUPPORT

Visit Az and Nina on the web:
www.giplan.com
A supportive site for anyone wanting to get into GI-eating by using the Simple GI Diet and motivational strategies. If you've already bought the book and need a quick inspirational fix or just some new menu ideas, this is worth a visit. For the uninitiated, the GI tips will whet your appetite.

www.thinkwelltobewell.com
Inspires you to check and challenge your thinking, approach and attitudes to food choices and many other aspects of life. It offers willpower boosters, diet tips, and a host of information on diet and diabetes.

Books
Think Well to Be Well by Azmina Govindji and Nina Puddefoot. Published by Diabetes Research & Wellness Foundation (2002).

Organizations
Registered dietitians hold the only legally recognizable graduate qualification in nutrition and dietetics. If you would like to find a dietitian near you, contact:

American Dietetic Association
120 South Riverside Plaza, Suite 2000
Chicago, IL 60606-6995

800-877-1600
www.eatright.org

General Health Websites
Healthy People 2010
www.healthypeople.gov
for ordering publications:
ODPHP Communications Support Center,
    P.O. Box 37366
Washington DC 20013-736
fax: 301-468-3028
This is a federal Health and Human Services program to improve the health of all people throughout the U.S. As they say it, "Healthy People 2010 challenges individuals, communities, and professionals—indeed, all of us—to take specific steps to ensure that good health, as well as long life, are enjoyed by all." A range of information and links to other sites are available online. They also provide written publications (list and order forms are online).

Active.com
www.active.com
888-543-7223 ext 4
A website that links you to all sorts of sports throughout the U.S., including individual sports, team sports, and park or community activities. A great resource for finding fun activities to meet your goal for physical activity.

INDEX

ABOUT THE AUTHORS

Azmina Govindji BSc RD is a consultant nutritionist and registered dietitian, broadcaster, best-selling author and Master NLP Practitioner.

She started her early career as a clinical dietitian in several hospitals (gaining direct experience with patients). She then spent eight years as the National Consultant on Diet and Diabetes when she was Chief Dietitian to Diabetes UK in Great Britain. This experience makes her particularly qualified to write this book, since GI is a concept that has been used in treating diabetes for years. She now runs her own practice providing dietetic consultancy to the food industry, healthcare professionals and the media. Her website is www.azminagovindji.com.

The author of 10 books, she lives in Great Britain.

Nina Puddefoot is a Master Practitioner and Certified NLP Trainer and development life coach. She works with cutting-edge models of thinking within multinational organizations and industries as well as individuals worldwide. Nina is a regular presenter of public programs, talks and workshops, and has been featured in a series about business and health on cable television in the UK.

Renowned for her ability to quickly establish relationships with sensitivity and humor, Nina strives to enrich and inspire the lives of others through her support for individuals' empowerment and passion.